THE TUBERCULOSIS SURVIVAL

HANDBOOK

2nd Edition

By

PAUL MAYHO

Foreword:
Richard Coker

Special Contributors:
Marcos Espinal, Ernesto Jaramillo

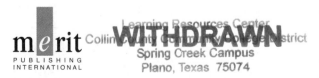

merit
PUBLISHING
INTERNATIONAL

Learning Resources Center
Collin County Community College District
WITHDRAWN
Spring Creek Campus
Plano, Texas 75074

Cover Design and Artwork by:

SMK Design

©2006 Merit Publishing International and Paul Mayho. All rights reserved. No part of this publication may be reproduced, stored in a retrieval system or transmitted in any form or by any means, electronic, mechanical, photocopying, recording or otherwise, without the prior permission of the copyright holder.

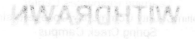

merit
PUBLISHING
INTERNATIONAL

THE TUBERCULOSIS SURVIVAL

HANDBOOK

2nd Edition

MERIT PUBLISHING INTERNATIONAL

European address:
50 Highpoint, Heath Road
Weybridge, Surrey KT13 8TP
England

Tel: (44) (0) 1932 844526
Fax: (44) (0) 1932 820419

North American address:
5840 Corporate Way, Suite 200
West Palm Beach, FL 33407
USA

Tel: 561 697 1116
Fax: 561 477 4961

Web: www.meritpublishing.com

ISBN: 978-1-873413-14-2
1-873413-14-9

In memory of Boris

CONTENTS

FOREWORD

Tuberculosis has probably been with us for as long as mankind has walked the earth. With improved socio-economic conditions in the affluent West along with access to effective treatment, TB disappeared from the public health radar screen in the latter decades of the twentieth century. Policy-makers', public health officials' and the public's attention were drawn to apparently more pressing problems. This was the case domestically and internationally. But TB had not disappeared. Indeed, in much of the world TB rates had remained high. But the West's attention was drawn elsewhere, as was the attention of the major multilateral institutions. By 1988, the World Health Organization had only one medical officer responsible for TB control at its Geneva headquarters. In the late 1980s and early 1990s, however, four factors converged to fuel the global epidemic, heighten public awareness, and engage political support for TB control.

The first was recognition that TB, while declining in affluent countries, was consistently not addressed in many developing countries. The second, was a dawning acknowledgement that affluent countries, through their domestic public health programs alone, could no longer remain immune from global epidemics. Globalization and the increased movements of people crossing countries were making more stark the frequent refrain that microbiological organisms do not respect borders. A third factor was the emergence of the HIV/AIDS epidemic and the complex interactions between HIV and TB. TB control is inextricably linked to HIV control. Globally, approximately 10% of all new cases of TB can be attributed to HIV.

A final factor was the sudden, sometimes unmanageable, outbreaks of Multidrug-resistant tuberculosis (MDR-TB). Major outbreaks in the late 1980s and early 1990s, notably in New York City, raised the specter of a potentially untreatable infectious disease transmitted casually, where anybody could be at risk. This latter issue also focused minds because of the costs incurred by both patients and public health authorities.

The confluence of these four factors made something of a mockery of earlier optimistic projections and plans for the eradication of TB drawn up in the 1980s. While aid for TB control was pitiful in the 1980s and early 1990s, this was to change. In 1990, for example, only 16 million in bilateral and multilateral support was made available to support global TB control efforts. Funding support now runs to billions of dollars each year, including support to control HIV. New institutions are committed to control and older institutions have expanded their portfolios into the health sphere.

The World Bank is now a major contributor to control efforts. The Global Fund to Fight AIDS, TB and Malaria (GFATM) and PEPFAR are new initiatives providing substantial sums and resources. Philanthropists such as Bill and Melinda Gates and George Soros have also made substantial contributions to enhance control. Allied to these disease specific responses, the global movement to respond effectively to the curse of poverty, in Africa especially (for example through the G8), means that the picture of global engagement on TB is very different from a decade ago.

Yet despite this global commitment to TB control, many people still, decades after the development of effective treatment, cannot access care and die from TB unnecessarily. And despite (or perhaps because) of the renewed energy and resources being dedicated to the global control of TB, the voices of one group are heard only rarely: people with TB.

Paul Mayho's excellent book goes a long way to making that voice louder. As Paul says, "The TB treatment journey is a long one and it is not only about taking pills." It is about the structures and systems that aid recovery. It is about the integration of health care systems with social support networks. It is about alleviating the economic and social barriers to access and care. It is about stopping the development of TB, a consequence of poverty, overcrowding, and malnutrition. Who knows this better than people who have had TB?

It is over a decade since Paul Mayho acquired MDR-TB. Paul had already been diagnosed with AIDS. At that time the outlook was extremely grim. Many people with AIDS who have also acquired MDR-TB succumbed within a month. Paul survived because of medical care he could access in the UK. He thrived because of his indomitable spirit and the support of his friends and colleagues. He also had important things to say. Some of these things are captured eloquently in this, the Second Edition, of *The Tuberculosis Survival Handbook*.

Dr. Richard Coker

Reader in Public Health
London School of Hygiene & Tropical Medicine

INTRODUCTION

Before the First Edition of *"The Tuberculosis Survival Handbook"* was
published in 1999, it was difficult to find a publisher. Publishers informed
me that it was not suitable because: "Tuberculosis has gone away, there is
no problem and there is no market." This is a common misconception and
was frustrating because many of us knew differently. In the light of the
responses received from publishers, I decided to self-publish and
ultimately, the book was a success. Merit Publishing International publishes
this *Second Edition* of *The Tuberculosis Survival Handbook* and I would like
to thank them for their recognition that tuberculosis is a growing problem
and the value this publication will bring to its readers.

Tuberculosis is a resurgent disease. Indeed, the World Health Organization
has gone as far as calling it a "global emergency"[1]. TB infects about
one-third of all humans worldwide. In 2005 alone, 9 million people were
diagnosed with the disease and more than 2 million died. About
40 million people have become latently infected with *Mycobacterium
tuberculosis* during 2005. About 80% of these new cases will have
occurred in just 22 countries and more than half are allocated to five
nations: Bangladesh, China, India, Indonesia, and Nigeria [2].

South East Asia has the largest number of cases and in Eastern Europe and
Africa the incidence of TB is rising. This is due mainly to the spread of
HIV/AIDS, the breakdown in global health services and the emergence of
Multidrug-resistant tuberculosis. Since 1992, progress has been made in
the United States to combat the disease, although 14,500 cases were
identified in the US alone in 2004 [2].

In the UK, there have been approximately 7,000 new cases of TB per year since the mid-1980s. Only five other countries in Europe have increasing TB rates: The Russian Federation, Ukraine, Romania, Kazakhstan and Uzbekistan.

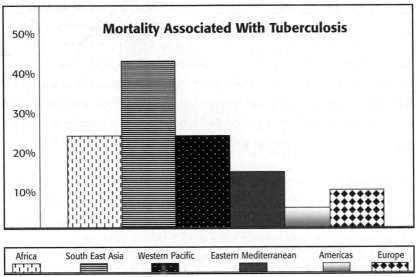

Mortality Associated With Tuberculosis

©WHO

MDR-TB (Multidrug-resistant TB) is a hugely growing problem. In 2003, the Stop TB Department in Geneva, Switzerland estimated that there were around 425,000 incident cases of MDR-TB worldwide. However, the actual prevalence of MDR-TB may be three times greater than its incidence. This could mean that the number of MDR-TB cases globally today could exceed one million[3].

Drug-resistant TB is transmitted in the same way as drug-susceptible TB. Primary resistance develops in persons initially infected with resistant organisms. Secondary resistance (acquired resistance) may develop during

TB therapy due to inadequate treatment regimen, not taking the prescribed regimen appropriately or using low quality medication.

Since the First Edition of this book was published, the global community has become much more aware of the problem posed by tuberculosis. It is now widely recognized that TB presents a threat to us all, but especially to the vulnerable members of society.

There is much information available for TB specialists in books and journals but very little for those that actually have the disease. When I experienced a rare form of tuberculosis in 1995, I felt lonely, alone and very frightened. There were no books available for the patient with TB to help them understand and deal with their condition.

The lack of information on TB for sufferers and the recognition of the importance of having information, became my motivation for writing this book. My aim with the First Edition - and now the Second - is to convey the message to those with tuberculosis that **'you are not alone'**.

The information in the new edition is written in simple terms, which makes it easy-to-read and understand. The text is very comprehensive; if you have tuberculosis or if you want a good understanding of TB and those living with it, you will find all you need to know about the disease in this publication. The book explains what happens and why to those with TB. Its other aim is to help guide readers through the TB treatment journey to the point in time when they will be cured. **There is the good news - Tuberculosis is a curable disease when it is treated and managed properly.**

Having had experience as both a health care worker and patient, I am in a unique position to write this book. I was formerly a student nurse but tested positive for HIV in 1990. After being diagnosed, I resigned from my training and worked as a volunteer in the HIV sector. I then wrote my first book, "Positive Carers", which was concerned with the rights and responsibilities of HIV-positive health care workers.

Shortly after completing the book, I was diagnosed with Multidrug-resistant tuberculosis (MDR-TB), a rare form of the disease. My life changed as dramatically as it did when I learned I was HIV-positive. This experience forced me to learn, very quickly, as much as I could about TB. Like me, some of those reading this book may fall into more than one category. Tuberculosis has no respect for profession, social status, color, creed or age: we are all vulnerable, but some more than others. Importantly, whether we are clinicians, health care workers or individuals with tuberculosis, we can all learn from one another to help improve our lives.

What makes this edition of *"The Tuberculosis Survival Handbook"* different to the First Edition? Apart from being completely restructured for easier reading and access, the text has also been updated with the most recent information and statistics available. In recognition that successfully treating tuberculosis requires a partnership between the care provider and patient, the text also includes a chapter on the clinician's perspective of TB. The chapter titled, *The Patient's Perspective* provides insight to timelines of TB from symptoms to diagnosis, medication, and finally, to being cured. Additionally, this chapter provides practical considerations and the important role that nurses play in relation to patients, particularly in terms of wellbeing, treatment and adherence to medication.

The last few years has seen many changes in the field of TB. The treatment model for TB is very traditional. For the most part, unlike HIV, there is a paternalistic approach to TB treatment and the emphasis rests with control. Slowly but surely, this is changing. Many TB specialists are coming around to the idea that treating and curing tuberculosis has to happen within the framework of a partnership between the health care provider and the patient, much like the management of HIV.

This book will be attractive to a wide audience of readers including patients, nurses, other healthcare providers, and medical students, and although the text has been written as simply as possible, several chapters are quite clinical. To aid the layperson to better understand the issues being discussed within the book, each chapter is concluded with an easy-to-read summary of what has been covered.

The popular "TB-Tips" that were in the First Edition have been grouped together for easier reference and can be found in Appendix A. Following these, there is a TB Treatment Chart as an extra aid to help readers through the TB treatment journey in Appendix B.

In summary, there is also a completely new final chapter that discusses the growing patient movement, which demands to be heard in order to play their role in TB control. This movement has been recognized at the highest level; engaging patients has become part of the World Health Organization's Stop TB Partnership's strategy for TB control [2]. For patients, if you have or have had tuberculosis, there are many opportunities for involvement and this chapter explains them.

There are many people to thank for their help in making this book a reality, all of whom recognized the need for a patient-led book. For their professional help, The Department of Health, especially Dr. Susan Turnbull & Dr. Jane Leese, Sherry Hussain, Division of Tuberculosis Elimination, CDC Atlanta, USA, Dr. Ian Everall at The Maudsley Hospital, London and Paul van Buynder of the Public Health Laboratory Service, London. Rosy Weston, Senior Pharmacist, for her input on pharmaceuticals and Jane Rowntree, Senior Dietician, for her nutritional advice, both also of St. Mary's Hospital, London. Gratitude also goes to Dr. Simon Magus for help with the First Edition.

An extra special thanks must go to Dr. Richard Coker, Dr. Marcos Espinal and Dr. Ernesto Jaramillo. Dr. Coker is author of *"From Chaos to Coercion"* and Reader in Public Health at the London School of Hygiene & Tropical Medicine. He is also the author of the Foreword for both editions and Medical Editor. Dr. Marcos Espinal of the Stop TB Partnership and Dr. Ernesto Jaramillo of the World Health Organization, both based in Geneva, Switzerland, are co-authors of "The Clinician's Perspective" in this publication. Thank you, also, Marcos, for being a friend and encouraging me in my work with TB. Also of the Stop TB Partnership, I would like to thank, Michael Luhan and Glenn Thomas, both within the Communications Department, for their support and friendship.

Other thanks to Ted Torfoss of LHL, Norway and Dr. Kitty Lambregst, KNVC, Netherlands. Case Gordon of TBTV.org, France for keeping me on my toes, Laura Hakokongas and Daniel Berman of the Campaign for Access to Essential Medicines (CAME) at Médecins Sans Frontières, Geneva, for giving me a chance (Laura, you taught me a lot!).

There are others for whom I have extra special gratitude without whose care, love and support I probably would not be here today. They are Russell Levy of Leigh Day & Co., London, AIDS pioneer John Campbell for sparking my will to fight all those years back, Terry White for his kindness and encouragement, Asha Pariagh, Miles Jones, Shay Costello, Steve Miller and everyone at the Environmental Health Department in the London Borough of Newham. Also, everyone at Balan's Café in Old Compton Street, London, for keeping the coffee coming!

Special thanks also goes to Robert Maynard for keeping my feet on the ground and the Hula-Hoops. Most importantly, I want to say thank you to the wonderful Mark King, for all the love and support he has shown me. Mark, sometimes you drive me nuts, but I could not have done any of this without you. You are my family.

Finally, I would like to say that I am always interested to hear about other people's experience of tuberculosis. If you would like to share your story with a wider audience or have any comments about this publication, please feel free to email me at **mystory@tbsurvivalproject.org** or visit *"The Tuberculosis Survival Project"* website at www.tbsurvivalproject.org.

Paul Mayho

Chapter 1

THE CLINICIAN'S PERSPECTIVE

Dr. Marcos Espinal, *Executive Secretary, Stop TB Partnership, World Health Organization Geneva, Switzerland.*

Dr. Ernesto Jaramillo, *Medical Officer. World Health Organization Geneva, Switzerland.*

Introduction

The World Health Organization (WHO) estimates that nearly 2 million people die with tuberculosis (TB) every year and almost 5,000 individuals every day [1]. The tragedy of TB affects mostly people of low and middle-income countries. Twenty-two countries, nine of them in Africa and eleven in Asia, are estimated to contribute 80% of the 9 million new cases of TB worldwide.

The paradox of such a human tragedy is that inexpensive tools to prevent, diagnose, treat, and cure TB have been available for decades. Individuals with coughs lasting more than two to three weeks should deliver at least two initial sputum samples to a laboratory performing smear microscopy examination for acid-fast bacilli (AFB). AFB represents either *Mycobacterium tuberculosis* or non-tuberculous *Mycobacteria*. If smear microscopy is positive for AFB in conjunction with clinical and radiological data, a diagnosis for TB is made.

Treatment will consist mainly of a combination of different drugs, which is to be taken over at least six months. This solution, as simple as it looks, is in fact a challenging experience for the individual affected. While they offer an answer to the problem, these tools are imperfect. Smear microscopy only detects 40-60% of individuals with TB. Drugs, although efficacious against TB, only

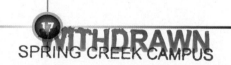
WITHDRAWN
SPRING CREEK CAMPUS

work if treatment is for at least six months and the individual is not infected with a drug-resistant strain of *Mycobacterium tuberculosis*. The vaccine currently in use is not efficacious against pulmonary TB, the most common form of disease.

In 1995, WHO drawing on the field experience of the International Union Against Tuberculosis and Lung Diseases (IUATLD) with the available tools[2], designed a public health strategy that contains all the essential elements to facilitate timely diagnosis and treatment to cure people with TB. The strategy, named DOTS, includes five essential actions to ensure its effectiveness[3]. More than 20 million people have been treated under DOTS since its introduction, and 182 countries have adopted it as national policy. Yet, despite all the progress achieved in the last several years, by the end of 2004, 47% of the estimated TB cases worldwide still did not have access to DOTS, and the global incidence of disease continues to grow at a rate of 1% per year[1].

DOTS is composed of five elements, all of which are essential to a successful TB control program outcome. These are:

1) Government commitment to make TB a priority program and to provide resources for nation-wide coverage.

2) Case detection from among persons with persistent cough mainly through sputum smear microscopy in a countrywide laboratory network.

3) An uninterrupted drug supply provided to health centres for the treatment of all TB patients.

4) Use of standardized short-course chemotherapy and a commitment of the patient and health worker to complete treatment ensuring that each dose of drug is taken.

5) A recording and reporting system for monitoring treatment outcome; cohort analysis to reach targets of 85% cure, and training and supervision to assure that this is accomplished.

Clinician and patient perspectives

Political, social, economic and biological forces drive the magnitude of the TB epidemic [4]. Therefore, a clinician's perspective cannot be presented in isolation without considering the multifactor genesis of the problem. In this chapter, we will present some of the issues a clinician has to face in his daily work interacting with the TB epidemic.

TB is not a difficult disease to treat. An individual with TB who is ready to admit he or she has a curable disease is on his or her way to achieve cure, provided a supportive environment is in place. Several situations come to mind. The first one is the complex patient, which very often has history of alcoholism, drugs, imprisonment, and family problems. These types of patients are usually not adherent with treatment and frequently abandon therapy. The approach to tackle the issue becomes a multidisciplinary one and the general practitioner would need the help of psychologists/psychiatrists, pneumologists, social workers, specialized nurses, and others. This is very often the case of patients affected with multidrug-resistant tuberculosis (MDR-TB), which is defined as resistance to at least isoniazid and rifampicin, the two most potent anti-TB drugs for patients with drug-susceptible TB.

MDR-TB is a major threat to TB control. The WHO estimates that 1 million people have MDR-TB and that 425,000 new MDR-TB cases occur every year [5]. The WHO/IUATLD Global Project on Anti-Tuberculosis Drug-Resistance Surveillance shows that drug-resistant TB is a widespread problem. In countries of Central Asia and Eastern Europe, TB simply cannot be controlled if MDR-TB is not properly addressed [6]. An important finding of this project is that the magnitude of drug-resistance is significantly correlated with the extent and misuse of anti-TB drugs. The more time the affected individual receives treatment without achieving cure, the more likely MDR-TB will occur.

Individuals with MDR-TB and general practitioners face tough decisions regarding the type of treatment to be used. Treatment for MDR-TB is at least 18 months, more expensive and adverse events can be more frequent and severe than that of drug-susceptible TB. Furthermore, for this type of disease, one or two treatment regimens do not fit all, as with the case of drug-susceptible TB for which two or three standardized treatment regimens are recommended. There is also evidence that costs of managing MDR-TB in industrialized countries could be as low as US$60,000 or as high as US$180,000 [7,8]. In resource-limited countries, evidence from pilot projects shows that the management of MDR-TB under programmatic conditions is feasible, effective and cost-effective when implemented in the context of a well-functioning DOTS program and based on specific WHO guidelines [9-10].

Another very common situation observed in resource-limited countries is the lack of respect for national policies by physicians who were trained in industrialized countries or physicians working in the private sector. Clinicians trained in industrialized low TB incidence countries are usually taught with non-applicable TB control policies to their less developed, high TB incidence countries. Such situations create a problem for the health system and patients. The applications of policies that are not relevant to resource-limited countries are detrimental to TB control and disrupt the health system.

There is a misconception in many resource-limited countries that government policies are not the best ones, nor are they for people who cannot afford proper treatment. Trained physicians usually learn the policies of the countries where they were trained. Patients are prescribed different treatment regimens, which are not in line with their own country's epidemiological situation and national policy. The public health implications of these policies are devastating, as this could be the beginning of a long road for an individual who could otherwise have been cured and instead, the threat of MDR-TB is very real for these patients.

Not unrelated to the above, is the emerging profitable private sector in several resource-limited countries in which many clinicians do their daily work. Countries with high TB incidence have to deal with a powerful private health care sector that is sometimes reluctant to use DOTS. This situation certainly contributes to derail national and global efforts[11]. Furthermore, the household economy of people with TB is greatly affected, as ill people keep moving from one general practitioner to another. A novel approach, called "public-private mix" is contributing to de-privatize the management of TB in such settings. The WHO defines the "public-private mix" as a collection of strategies linking all healthcare providers within the private and public sectors to national tuberculosis programs for expansion of the DOTS strategy[11]. Preliminary reports indicate that "public-private mix" is feasible and effective to manage TB in the private sector[12].

The HIV crisis is the biggest challenge the TB epidemic faces and both physicians and patients must face this grim reality. It is estimated that nearly 13% of the estimated 8.9 million new cases of TB in 2004 were HIV infected[1]. However, in Africa 33% of the estimated TB cases are infected with HIV. TB is the leading killer among HIV-infected people with weakened immune systems; overall, 250,000 TB deaths are HIV-associated, most of which are in Africa. Health care systems in Africa have been seriously impacted by the HIV epidemic. Physicians and patients are experiencing several difficulties and constraints to provide and receive proper care for TB. Physicians' constraints include lack of job stability, which steer a great deal of migration to better paid jobs in industrialized countries, lack of incentives and stimulation to continue fighting the TB epidemic, poor training, and weak infrastructure.

The Stop TB Partnership has placed Africa as top priority to address the dual effect of HIV and TB. Several initiatives are under way, including the implementation of a blueprint for rapid action following the declaration of TB as an emergency by the Ministers of Health of African countries in 2005, collaboration with the WHO-based global health workforce alliance to address the massive human workforce crisis that is currently taking place, and jointly working with several partners and other initiatives to strengthen health systems.

For African patients, the lack of access to DOTS' services is a critical problem. Long distances to health posts make people unable to access proper care. Anti-retroviral drugs are still in need of greater deployment in Africa, and only a limited number of HIV-infected patients are accessing this vital therapy. Also, palliative care for HIV-infected people with TB is not widely available. The Stop TB Partnership, through its working group on TB/HIV led by the WHO, has issued guidelines and recommendations for joint collaborative measures between HIV and TB national programs [13]. If implemented, these guidelines could help to alleviate the burden of HIV-related TB. Close collaboration between the HIV and TB control programs will facilitate the provision of a synergistic response by the health system to people affected by both epidemics.

A new strategy to tackle recalcitrant threats to TB control
The time to accelerate efforts to ensure current diagnostic and therapeutic tools reach all those in need, and mainly the poor, has come and should be treated as a priority. But also, development of new tools

including diagnostics, drugs, and vaccines should be a top priority. In 2006, the Stop TB Partnership launched the most ambitious, though realistic, global plan to date to accelerate efforts to control TB globally, to tackle major threats to the progress achieved so far, and to put in place new tools to replace the old tools [14].

The 10-year Global Plan is a comprehensive, inclusive, blueprint of actions to reach the 2015 Millennium Development Goals to halve incidence of TB and start the reversal of this human disaster. The Plan needs to be implemented by countries, international agencies, academia, communities affected by the disease, and the scientific community. The implementation of the Global Plan actions provided is funded and will set the path for the elimination of TB as a public health problem by 2050.

The Plan will be implemented through the new WHO Stop TB strategy, which has been endorsed by the Stop TB Partnership. The new strategy acknowledges that control of TB requires a more comprehensive approach to address obstacles impeding further expansion in quality and quantity of sound TB control. This new strategy has two important goals: 1) Reduction of the global burden of TB in line with the Millennium Development Goals and achievement of universal access to high-quality diagnosis and patient-centered treatment by reducing the human suffering and socio-economic burden associated with TB, protecting the poor and vulnerable populations from TB, TB/HIV and multidrug-resistant TB, and 2) Supporting the development of new tools and enabling their timely and effective use.

STOP TB STRATEGY

1. Pursue high-quality DOTS expansion and enhancement
   - Political commitment with increased and sustained financing
   - Case detection through quality-assured bacteriology
   - Standardized treatment with supervision and patient support
   - An effective drug supply and management system
   - Monitoring and evaluation system, and impact measurement

2. Address TB/HIV, MDR-TB and other challenges
   - Implement collaborative TB/HIV activities
   - Prevent and control multidrug-resistant TB
   - Address prisoners, refugees and other high-risk groups and special situations

3. Contribute to health system strengthening
   - Actively participate in efforts to improve system-financing, management, service delivery and the workforce crisis
   - Share innovations that strengthen systems, the Practical Approach to Lung Health (PAL)
   - Adapt innovations from other fields

4. Engage all care providers
   - Public-Public, and Public-Private Mix (PPM)
   - International Standards for Tuberculosis Care

5. Empower people with TB, and communities
   - Advocacy, communication and social mobilization
   - Community participation in TB care
   - Patients' Charter for Tuberculosis Care

6. Enable and promote research
   - Program based operational research
   - Research to develop new diagnostics, drugs and vaccines

Summary

Physicians providing care for TB, nurses, and patients with the disease are facing tough challenges to conquer a pandemic that is ravaging the world. They are the most critical players to conquer TB, a disease that has been with us since the time of the pharaohs, a total embarrassment for the international community.

While the current tools are not perfect, they still do the job and sound policy recommendations are available to prevent, diagnose, treat, and cure TB based on these tools. Patients should consult others if doubts arise about the type of care they have been provided. These include local agencies, medical societies, Ministries of Health, international agencies such as the WHO, IUATLD, and the Stop TB Partnership. Likewise, physicians should do the same and not think they have the ultimate knowledge, a situation that is quite common in resource-limited countries. Blaming patients for defaulting treatment is not correct behavior, as the ultimate responsibility is with the provider.

The time for new tools will come in due course. It is expected that by 2015 new tools will be in place to facilitate better care for the people affected by TB. These tools will be the first step for the elimination of TB by 2050. Conquering TB is possible: let us not lose hope, we can make it.

Chapter 2

A PATIENT'S PERSPECTIVE

"Like Paul Mayho, John Keats, the Brönte sisters, Chekhov, George Orwell, and millions of others unknown have had tuberculosis. They, unlike Paul but like millions each year even now, died from their disease. Yet what separates Paul and his contemporaries is that tuberculosis need no longer be a "death warrant". Effective treatment is available today and has been so for several decades" [1].

Dr. Richard Coker, From Chaos to Coercion, St. Martins Press

In 1990, I was diagnosed HIV-positive. By 1995, I became ill with AIDS and frequently was required to stay in a hospital for short periods of time. On one of those occasions, I had been admitted for investigations into a possible gastro-intestinal infection. Unfortunately, I was to come away from the hospital with much more than doctors had thought; I had been infected with a rare form of tuberculosis, which was resistant to usual TB treatment. It was called Multidrug-resistant tuberculosis or MDR-TB.

At the time I was ill, in April 1995, there had been another young man in the hospital with MDR-TB. This disease is highly contagious and it had been transmitted to me and to others, due to poor infection control (the case is well documented and can be researched by typing my surname into an Internet search engine).

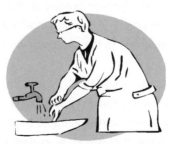

At the time I was infected with MDR-TB, I had been working as a volunteer with an HIV/AIDS organization in London. This reinforced the view that it is better to stay busy than allow oneself to dwell too much on an illness. Work was a catharsis and helped to keep me going up until that point in time. Increasingly, however, I was becoming weaker. As I worked, the TB bacilli was replicating slowly inside my lungs. By the end of June that year, I was experiencing chest pain that felt unusual, as if the outside of my lungs was being rubbed with something abrasive within my rib cage.

Gradually, I became more fatigued and developed a creeping temperature intermittently and mainly at night. The chest pains, which had until then been occasional, began to feel more constant and knowing I had an infection, but not knowing the cause. I once again went to the hospital. In hospital, a chest X-ray was taken and a sputum (phlegm) sample. I did go home afterward and even with the temperature, chest pain and fatigue, tried to get on with my life.

It was late July by now, one month later, when I returned to the hospital for a check-up. I had not had a result from the hospital about the sputum test and naturally assumed that my symptoms could not have been too serious. I spoke again with the doctor and told him that I still felt a slightly unwell but increasingly tired. However, as I was finishing my first book at the time and regularly working late into the night, I had attributed the tiredness to long hours of work. With no answers, I again left the hospital.

On 27th July 1995, I wrote the final page of my first book. Three years of research and work was coming to an end and I felt tearful. However, that day for me was going to be remembered in the future for entirely different reasons. My ex-partner rang to say that the hospital was trying to urgently contact me. I telephoned the doctor and he told me to go to the hospital immediately where he would meet me. On arrival, the doctor informed me something had grown in the sputum sample given to them some weeks earlier. The incubated sample had grown bacteria that could be tuberculosis.

I was placed alone in a side-room in the hospital. On occasions when nurses came into the room, I asked questions but none of them seemed to be able to provide answers. I was feeling almost detached from reality at this point, as if this experience was not happening to me and I was watching someone else's life unfold. Eventually, the doctor came in and tried to explain what was happening. I was frightened. Having HIV is one thing but Tuberculosis was quite another. HIV is transmissible sexually, for the most part. As long as certain precautions are taken and common sense applied, there is little risk of transmitting the virus to others. Tuberculosis, however, is an airborne bacterial infection. I wondered if I had infected anyone else and I also wondered who had infected me.

I was requested to make a list of all of the people I had been in contact with since the previous April when last in hospital. This is called 'contact tracing' and it was done to ensure that I had not, or learn whether I had, infected anyone else. My mind raced; I had been to many places and had been in contact with many people. In addition to work, I had been in restaurants, public transportation, and even had a holiday. I felt embarrassed about what other people would think of me when they found out that I might have infected them with TB.

I was moved to a negative-pressure isolation room. This is a room with an ante-chamber where the air pressure inside is lower than the room outside. It is a system that prevents any bacteria escaping out to the rest of the hospital. I wondered what 'isolation' meant and the doctor was unable to tell me how long I might be there. Did it mean that I could not see anyone at all? Would I ever be able to leave the room again?

The walls of the isolation room were bare and the room had no curtains. It is standard infection control procedure to take curtains down once the previous person has vacated the room. I was told a new set would arrive soon but I wondered whether they would. Worrying about whether or not I would have curtains seems a little strange in retrospect, considering what was happening to me but I was confused and frightened. I needed explanations but when the doctor tried to provide them, I did not seem to be able to retain the information. Those that came into the room had to wear masks to prevent them from breathing in the bacteria that might be in the air and this added to the increasingly surreal experience.

The days began to blend into one another. I found it difficult to keep track of events and started to keep a diary as an aid. Sometimes when I slept, I would dream I had been outside of the room but I would wake up and find myself back again. Freedom seemed to exist only in my dreams and writing.

I was started on TB medication as a pre-emptive measure while more tests were undertaken to confirm the diagnosis. It took quite some time for the new test results to come back and the nurses kept saying that they would "come tomorrow", but "tomorrow" never seemed to come. I had provided another sputum sample to look for TB bacilli, which they called a 'sputum smear' test. When the result came back, it was negative. Although this was good news, it was not conclusive. I was informed that a sample would need to be incubated to see if anything, not instantly visible, would grow over time. This is called a 'sputum culture'. Eventually, the test came back and it was also negative. All appeared to be well.

Although I was allowed to go home, I was told that as a precaution I had to try and limit contact with others. Frankly, I could not understand that if the tests were negative, why I must stay away from people. I now understand the reason for being cautioned: TB replicates very slowly and can take time to become visible in sputum smear and culture tests.

After all I had been through, I finally decided to seek a second opinion. When I met with my new doctor, he undertook more tests and decided it would be sensible as a precautionary measure to re-admit me once again to the hospital. Once again, I found myself in another isolation room, which was much like the other. I began having drenching, night sweats, which is another symptom of TB. I waited for news and wondered whether or not I actually had tuberculosis. With the symptoms that I was experiencing, it was beginning to look more likely and a few days later I received the news I had been dreading.

A group of physicians came to see me with the results of my most recent sputum culture. I did have tuberculosis, but it was a more serious than originally thought. It was not 'standard' TB; I had contracted Multidrug-resistant tuberculosis, otherwise known as MDR-TB. MDR-TB is much more difficult to treat than tuberculosis that is fully drug-sensitive because it is resistant to drugs that are usually used to treat it.

I was started on medication for MDR-TB called 'second-line' drugs. Often these drugs take longer to work and have more unpleasant side effects than the normally used 'first-line' drugs.

Within a short period of time, other 'sputum smear' tests showed that I was actively expelling TB bacteria when I coughed and this indicated that I was infectious. As the TB bacteria multiplied in my lungs, I began to get very ill. The cough progressively worsened and on occasion there were small specks of blood in it, I was losing weight, looking bad and feeling terrible.

If I was to be cured of this disease, it was vital to take all medications correctly. The person who had passed MDR-TB to me would have started with fully drug-sensitive TB. However, it was possible that he had not taken his medication properly and the bacteria had adapted to the first-line drugs. Subsequently, the TB might have become a drug-resistant strain by the time that it was passed to me.

With every dose of the TB medication, a nurse would watch me take the pills to ensure I was adherent. Although it was not a nice feeling to be observed, it was necessary. If I did not take the medication properly, I would not be cured and the TB bacilli could become even more resistant to the drugs.

Isolation was a horrible experience but not everyone must go through it. There was concern about my particular condition because it was drug-resistant and that was why it was necessary. Personally, it was a very lonely experience in the isolation room and it was increasingly strange to have people communicating with me while wearing a mask. I missed human contact.

The doctors involved did not know whether I was going to survive and frankly, I had my doubts. It was rare to have someone with HIV and MDR-TB at the same time and even my doctor had not previously come across it. It was, of course, very difficult to deal with the possibility of dying.

I considered whether the last place I saw would be the ceiling of the isolation room with eyes peering at me over orange masks. This was not an experience I would ever want to go through again.

I maintained the medication schedule and gradually started to improve. My energy levels started to rise and I began to gain weight. Mentally, it was important to be as constructive as possible with my time so I wrote quite a bit. As I felt stronger I began to exercise with sit-ups and press-ups. I requested an exercise bike and weights and I even ordered a sun-bed to be delivered to the room! Three months passed and by the time I was discharged, I looked better than ever!

As a result of taking all of the TB medication, I started to produce negative test results. I was not cured but I was no longer infectious, nor a risk to others. I was finally allowed to go home.

Fortunately, the contact tracing exercise was negative and I did not appear to have infected anyone else. I remained on TB medication for nearly two and half years. I was also required to 'check-in' with nurses at a local health center for Directly Observed Therapy (DOT), which helped to monitor my progress with the TB treatment.

Eventually, I was cured and it has now been over 10 years since I developed MDR-TB. Today my life is very different and I am well - one would not even know that I ever had the disease. I was one of the fortunate cases. MDR-TB is expensive to treat and many countries cannot afford second-line drugs. Sadly, in some countries many people with tuberculosis do die. Yet, we have a cure for TB.

So, why do so many people die of the disease? There are several reasons attributed to the TB death rate: non-adherence to treatment, the length of time it takes to complete the treatment, and the degree of commitment required to take the medication. In some parts of the world, there is also a problem with access to TB treatment. Patients can be cured of tuberculosis wherever there is access to treatment and providing the medication is taken correctly. Patients must only stop taking the medication when told to do so by a TB specialist.

There is no secret contained in these pages as to how to survive the disease. **It is all about adherence to the medication.** This book will help you understand TB, how it is diagnosed and treated. It also contains some strategies to help with the TB treatment journey and for patients this book will help you to realize that you are not alone.

Chapter 3

WHAT IS TUBERCULOSIS ?

"Tuberculosis is on the increase and is responsible for the deaths of more than two million people a year"

The World Health Organization

Tuberculosis is a contagious disease. A type of bacteria called *Mycobacterium tuberculosis* or *M. tuberculosis* causes it. Bacteria are tiny organisms that reproduce by dividing, and can be shaped like a sphere, rod or spiral. They are present virtually everywhere. Some of them are harmless - others are very dangerous. The dictionary definition of a mycobacterium is: "a Gram-positive rod like genus of aerobic bacteria, some species of which are harmful to man"[1].

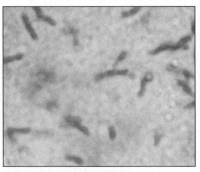
Rod-shaped mycobacterium

"Tuberculosis is an infectious disease that usually attacks the lungs but TB can attack almost any part of the body. It is spread from person to person through the air. When people with TB in their lungs (called 'pulmonary tuberculosis') cough, laugh, sneeze, sing, or even talk, the germs that spread TB may be spread into the air. If another person breathes in the germs there is a chance that they will become infected with tuberculosis"[2].

Left untreated, or not treated properly, tuberculosis can kill. In 1998, a WHO Fact Sheet on TB stated, "Tuberculosis kills more youth and adults than any other infectious disease in the world today. It is a bigger killer than malaria and AIDS combined, and kills more women each year than all the combined causes of maternal mortality. It also kills 100,000 children each year"[3]. The good news is that tuberculosis is a disease that we know a lot about and can cure... if it is treated properly.

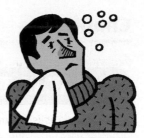
Tuberculosis germs are airborne

Multidrug-resistant tuberculosis (MDR-TB) is a type of TB that quite often develops in patients that do not complete the proper treatment for TB. Without proper treatment, 'super' resistant strains could occur for which there is currently no cure.

Tuberculosis: The Past

The story of tuberculosis puts fiction to shame. It may surprise many to know that tuberculosis is "probably as old as the earth itself - surviving in the primeval mud at the very beginning of time"[4]. Archaeological evidence of tuberculosis has been found in fossilized bones. Hippocrates (460-375 BC), the Greek physician, called the disease 'phthisis', a term formerly applied to many wasting diseases and connected with the lungs. He probably called it this for the same reason that it was called 'consumption' many centuries later. The disease, as we shall find out later, occasionally causes dramatic weight loss. Strangely, this look was thought to be attractive in the eighteenth and nineteenth centuries! The consumptive poet was something of an icon in the art world. The disease had curious romantic associations. Indeed, some people still hold this romantic notion of the disease and think of it in this historical context. Far from being a disease of the past, tuberculosis is resurgent.

TB can affect not just the lungs but also almost any part of the body. A few hundred years ago, one of the most common occurrences was the bacterium attacking the lymph glands, often in the neck. This was given the name 'scrofula', but was often called the 'King's Evil', because of the widely held belief that the touch of a royal hand would cure the afflicted person [5]. In 1720, the English physician, Benjamin Marten published *"A New Theory of Consumption."* He described the disease as being caused by "wonderfully minute living creatures"[6]. This was very forward thinking, as the bacterium was not officially discovered until 160 years later.

The scientist, Dr. Robert Koch, first suspected the mode of TB transmission. He recognized that most cases seemed to begin in the respiratory tract (the lungs and throat) and were therefore likely to be exhaled [7]. In 1882, the doctor announced the discovery of a staining technique that enabled the visualization of *Mycobacterium tuberculosis* under the microscope for the first time.

'Staining' means the use of dye to color tissues or micro-organisms so they are easier to view for examination. Once stained, most bacteria decolorize with acid. Mycobacterium retains the stain and is, therefore, called 'acid fast'; Subsequently, Mycobacteria are known as the 'acid fast bacilli' (AFB). The discovery heralded a new and exciting era in medicine. Once the bacteria had been identified, it seemed that the battle could begin properly against this age-old adversary.

In the United States, concern about the spread of tuberculosis played a role in the movement to prohibit public spitting, except into spitoons. In Europe, deaths from TB fell from 500 out of 100,000 in 1850 to 50 out of 100,000 by 1950[8]. Improvements in public health were reducing tuberculosis even

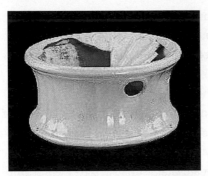

U.S. made 19th century yellow ware spittoon from Five Points, New York City

before the arrival of antibiotics, although the disease's significance was still such that when the Medical Research Council was formed in Britain in 1913 its first project was tuberculosis.

Another important development was the discovery by Doctors Calmette and Guerin of a 'tamed' living bacterium[9]. The word, 'tamed' is used in the sense that it was not particularly harmful and it created the basis for a vaccine called BCG ("Bacille Calmette-Guerin"). BCG vaccine is one of the most widely used vaccines in the world and is currently given at or soon after birth to children in over 100 countries to minimize the potential for serious forms of TB disease [27].

During the Second World War, the most powerful weapons against tuberculosis were developed: the chemotherapeutic agents. Thereafter followed a stream of such treatments used to fight TB.

Tuberculosis: The Present
In 1996, A. Karlen stated, "An alarming tide of new and resurgent diseases has been rising around the world for decades. Now it advances further than ever. This signals a crisis in the history of the human species. We have brought it on by rending the fabric of our environment, changing our behavior, and ironically, by our inventiveness in increasing the length and quality of our lives - Ignorance is a destructive luxury when infections threaten to take more lives than war and famine"[10]. Diseases once thought conquered by medical science are returning. Slowly but surely the rosy

future presented by the wonder of antibiotics is beginning to collapse [11]. Antibiotics have only been around for about 60 years and unfortunately the weaknesses of this relatively new development are already becoming apparent.

There is little doubt that antibiotics were a wonderful discovery but it is their indiscriminate use, which has caused the problem [12]. Many diseases, which we thought were moving towards eradication due to antibiotics have begun to resist our greatest ally. The bacteria are more sophisticated than originally thought and like any living organism, they have to reproduce to secure their survival. Therefore, to ensure their own survival, they are learning how to survive the antibiotics we use against them.

As previously mentioned, one reason for the return of TB is the organism's ability to adapt, so that some drugs used to attack it become ineffectual. TB then takes on its Multidrug-resistant form. Another reason for TB's return is the ease with which people can now travel globally, taking the disease with them from areas of high prevalence. This is, of course, due to wider-reaching, more efficient transport systems coupled with greater freedom of movement created by the opening of political borders.

In the document titled, *The Interdepartmental Working Group on Tuberculosis*, produced by the UK Department of Health in September 1998, we see that "The incidence of tuberculosis in the UK was at its highest at the beginning of the 19th century. It had fallen considerably, even before the introduction of specific anti-tuberculosis measures such as chemotherapy (in the 1940s) and BCG immunization (in the 1950s) helped to hasten the decline.

Some slowing of the decline occurred in the 1960s, in association with substantial immigration from parts of the world with high rates of tuberculosis such as the Indian sub-continent, although the incidence in the majority of the white population continued to decline... several factors are thought to have contributed including demographic changes (especially an aging population), continued high rates of tuberculosis among new immigrants and the effects of poverty and homelessness, as well as, to a relatively small extent, the HIV epidemic"[13].

Man and micro-organisms have always been in conflict. One can see that throughout history, there are as many failures as victories. The past 50 years have proven the most successful but the next 50 years may describe a different story. Alarmingly, some scientists claim that the early 21st century will be more reminiscent of the Middle Ages in terms of disease [14]. There are many previously unknown diseases, such as AIDS, Lassa fever, and the disease caused by the Ebola virus emerging alongside newly returning diseases such as tuberculosis.

Some notable comparisons may be made between tuberculosis and other diseases with regard to resistance to treatment with antibiotics. However, unlike AIDS, Lassa and Ebola, tuberculosis is a disease that we know quite a lot about. It is "man's rending of the fabric of our environment" [15] that has sadly caused the problems we now face with regard to the increase in incidence of tuberculosis. Unfortunately, we have allowed the disease to return.

Tuberculosis: The Future
Since the introduction of anti-tubercular treatments, initially, the number of reported cases steadily declined. The figures on all reported cases produced by the Public Health Laboratory Service for England and Wales have clearly shown this. Worryingly, this is no longer the trend. Since 1985, the number of reported cases has plateaued with little fluctuation. There seems to be

little difference between the figures produced for 1985 and those for 1997. Twelve years of constant fighting against the disease should have produced a further decline in its incidence but this has not been the case.

In a press release in 1993, The World Health Organization declared that TB was presenting a "global emergency". The disease was returning and without prompt action, the problem threatened to spiral out of control [16]. Although the trend mentioned in the paragraph above is based on UK data, it is indicative of the global situation. For example, 10 to 15 million people in the United States are infected with TB and could develop TB disease in future [17]. In other parts of the world, such as Africa and Asia, the growing incidence of tuberculosis is startling (see figures in the Introduction).

Estimated TB incidence and mortality, 2003						
	Number of cases (thousands)		Cases per 100 000 population		Deaths from TB (including TB deaths in people infected with HIV)	
WHO region	All forms (%)	Smear-positive	All forms	Smear-positive	Number (thousands)	Per 100 000 population
Africa	2372 (27)	1013	345	147	538	78
The Americas	370 (4)	165	43	19	54	6
Eastern Mediterranean	634 (7)	285	122	55	144	28
Europe	439 (5)	196	50	22	67	8
South-East Asia	3062 (35)	1370	190	85	617	38
Western Pacific	1933 (22)	868	112	50	327	19
Global	8810 (100)	3897	140	62	1747	28

©http://www.who.int/mediacentre/factsheets/fs104/en/

In another press release issued by the World Health Organization in March 1998, it was estimated that "between now and 2020, nearly one billion more people will be newly infected, 200 million people will get sick, and

70 million will die from TB - If control is not strengthened"[18]. When a statement like this is made by such a respected organization, it is clear that TB is a problem that cannot be ignored.

TB infection and TB disease - is there a difference?
To fully comprehend tuberculosis, it is important to understand that there is a difference between latent TB infection and active TB disease.

Latent TB Infection
It is quite possible to be infected with the TB bacteria, but not be ill or infectious. This is called "latent infection". The World Health Organization estimates that a third of the world's population, two billion worldwide, is latently infected. Most people who are latently infected will never become ill with TB and it is estimated that only 10% of those latently infected will go on to develop active TB disease [18]. Normally, the immune system can trap the bacteria and prevent it from making one ill. Essentially, the bacteria lies dormant and in most cases will never evolve.

It must be remembered that each day we come into contact with thousands of different types of bacteria. However, sometimes organisms break away from the trap set by the immune system and start to replicate (some reasons why this might occur are discussed later in this chapter). When this occurs, the active TB disease can develop. Left untreated, active TB disease can kill and is a danger to others. Latent TB infection alone simply means that at some point, one has come across bacteria that cause TB; it does not make one ill and is not a danger to others.

Active TB Disease
When active TB disease occurs, it can show anywhere in the body. Most commonly, it occurs in the lungs. This is called pulmonary tuberculosis.

When TB occurs anywhere else in the body, it is called extra-pulmonary tuberculosis. As TB is an airborne disease, it needs to be exhaled by someone who has active disease. Therefore, if a person has TB elsewhere in the body other than the lungs, they cannot be infectious since it cannot be exhaled. This does not mean, of course, that extra-pulmonary TB is less dangerous to the individual who has it. It does not matter where the disease resides. Both pulmonary and extra-pulmonary TB when left untreated can cause much damage and potentially kill. It should also be remembered that it is possible for bacteria residing elsewhere in the body to travel to the lungs, thereby making the person infectious. It is equally important that both pulmonary and extra-pulmonary TB are treated.

The Difference Between Latent TB Infection and Active Pulmonary TB Disease	
A Person with Latent TB Infection	**A Person with Active TB Disease**
	Has symptoms that may include:
• Has no symptoms • Does not feel sick • Cannot spread TB to others • Has a normal chest x-ray and sputum test.	• A bad cough that lasts 3 weeks or longer • Pain in the chest • Coughing up blood or sputum • Weakness or fatigue • Weight loss • No appetite • Chills • Fever • Sweating at night • May spread TB to others • May have an abnormal chest X-ray, or positive sputum smear or culture.

©National Center for HIV, STD and TB Prevention: Division of Tuberculosis Prevention

What are the symptoms of TB?

The symptoms of TB can manifest in a variety of ways, but few people will have all of the symptoms mentioned here. It is important to see a doctor immediately if you develop these symptoms, particularly if you have had TB before or are known to be latently infected. If you are already on TB medication and these symptoms develop, you should tell your TB specialist. The medication you are taking may not be working properly, and the clinician may need to adjust or change the drugs.

If you develop active TB disease you may:

- Suffer from fatigue
- Begin to lose weight
- Have loss of appetite
- Develop a fever
- Experience heavy night sweats
- Have swollen glands
- With pulmonary TB you may get any of the symptoms above accompanied by a cough. You may have chest pain and might be coughing up blood or blood stained sputum (phlegm). The medical term for coughing up blood is 'hemoptysis'. You may also feel short of breath.
- With extra-pulmonary TB, the symptoms will be based upon the part of the body affected. For example, TB of the lymph node will be characterized by severe swelling of the gland, spinal TB will be characterized by pain and impaired mobility, TB meningitis will present with neurological dysfunction, such as headache. As extra-pulmonary TB does not occur in the lungs, there is unlikely to be a cough. However the symptoms of fever, fatigue, loss of appetite and weight loss are usually present.

The onset of the symptoms of active TB disease can be very slow and insidious because the bacteria replicate very slowly and can take quite some time for one to become ill. You may not get all of the symptoms delineated above but none of them should be ignored. Certainly if a cough persists for more than three weeks or any of the other symptoms listed above are in evidence, a medical opinion should be sought. If you are on treatment for TB already then you should not wait, but present to the doctor immediately to ensure the medication is working properly.

Who can get tuberculosis?

We have already established that TB is an airborne disease and it is important to realize that anyone can be latently infected with tuberculosis. Although many of us may already be infected, some people are at higher risk of going on to develop active TB disease. Let us look at the factors that influence transmission of latent TB infection and why some people develop active TB disease.

People who share the same breathing space

Certainly the duration of exposure is important. The risk to the general population increases significantly the longer someone who is infectious with the disease stays unidentified and/or untreated for the infection. The longer one is around someone with infectious tuberculosis, the higher the risk of becoming infected [20]. More prolonged and sustained contact is also a factor that could potentially lead to latent infection becoming active TB disease because the immune system becomes overwhelmed with the amount of bacteria to which it is being exposed [21].

Most infections occur in settings where people are in regular close contact. For example, clusters of TB disease are often found within families or those that share accommodation. This also includes institutions such as prisons, hospitals and nursing homes [22]. The incidence of TB is higher in urban areas rather than rural ones. This is simply because the way of life in cities presents more opportunity for contact. In rural settings, there is less opportunity for contact and therefore, fewer cases of the disease. The risk of transmission of infection increases with population density [23].

People living in warm climates that spend more time outdoors have less exposure to tuberculosis because the bacteria disperse rapidly outdoors. People living in colder climates are at greater risk of infection due to poor air circulation in closed environments, such as where there are closed windows and doors. In geographical areas where there are long cold winters and people congregate indoors, there is more opportunity for exposure to the tuberculosis bacteria through prolonged and sustained contact [24].

People who already have health or social problems
Although latent TB infection is contained by the immune system, rendering the bacteria inactive, an individual may have been previously exposed to the bacteria, be latently infected and then develop active TB disease years later. This can happen for a variety of health and social reasons.

Poverty is one of the main drivers of active TB disease. If people cannot afford to eat, they are not going to have healthy immune systems that keep tuberculosis at bay. Good nutrition is vital to maintaining health. Social problems such as homelessness, poor and overcrowded living conditions, alcoholism and the use of illegal drugs are also factors. All of these factors and others can have an impact on the general standard of our health and how the immune system responds to latent TB infection.

Other people at risk are those with health problems affecting the immune system such as HIV/AIDS, diabetes, certain cancers and people taking drugs for other existing medical conditions. When the immune system is not working at its optimum level, it cannot prevent latent TB infection becoming active TB disease.

Multidrug-resistant tuberculosis

The history of tuberculosis shows that some bacteria have become resistant to drugs used to treat the disease. The emergence of drug-resistant bacteria has been observed since antibiotics were first discovered and widely used. "In the case of tuberculosis it very quickly became evident that resistance to TB treatment rapidly emerged unless a combination of anti-tuberculosis drugs was used "[25].

As scientists strive to develop cures and to conquer disease, it is unlikely that they will ever succeed in eradicating all harmful organisms from the environment. Indeed, just as we were getting used to the idea of effective control over bacterial infection through the miracle of antibiotics, there is growing evidence of more virulent strains of bacteria that have genetically acquired resistance to multiple drugs. For example, in the US a strain of tuberculosis has been observed which is resistant to virtually all the available antibiotics. A relationship based on an inter-dependency between humans and micro-organisms exists, with one achieving dominance over the other [26].

Strains of tuberculosis, resistant to the two main first-line drugs, isoniazid and rifampicin, is termed 'Multidrug-resistant tuberculosis' (MDR-TB). It is conceivable that in time, some strains of tuberculosis could become resistant to all of the drugs used against it, potentially creating an incurable "super-bug" [27].

NEW CASES OF MDR-TB IN 2000	
• Russian Federation	5,864
• The Philippines	7,642
• Pakistan	26,201
• India	63,136
• China	68,364

The World Health Organization estimates that up to 50 million persons worldwide may be infected with drug resistant strains of TB. Also, 425,000 new cases of MDR-TB are diagnosed around the world each year and 79% of the MDR-TB cases now show resistance to three or more drugs.

Drug-resistance can occur for a number of reasons. An individual can come into contact with an already drug-resistant strain and subsequently develop MDR-TB, or a patient may have fully drug-sensitive tuberculosis but demonstrate drug-resistance during a course of treatment that is either inadequate, or incomplete.

Farmers who use pesticides on their fields will tell you that every few of years they have to change the pesticide they use to prevent resistance developing among the pests. In the same way, tuberculosis may develop resistance to drugs. In cases where it has not been completely eradicated by treatment, for example when a patient has not taken medication at the appropriate times, any remaining bacteria may develop resistance. If this happens, the patient may pass on a drug-resistant strain.

This process is repeated endlessly, with drug-resistant strains passing from person to person, failure to take medication appropriately, and the disease 'learning' how to adapt to different drugs. Potentially, there is the frightening scenario where TB strains completely resistant to all medication emerge, and circulate among the population as a whole. Taking medication correctly is one way in which this may be prevented.

Tuberculosis and HIV Co-infection

Incidence data shows that large numbers of the world's population are latently infected with TB. In other words, although the TB bacteria are present in the body, the disease does not develop, remaining 'dormant'. If for any reason the immune system is weakened, the bacteria are no longer held in check, and active TB disease can develop. This is typically the case of people with HIV.

Tuberculosis is, for the most part, a treatable and curable disease. HIV is becoming more manageable but at present is not curable. I have heard some people refer to being co-infected with TB and HIV as "the Devil's Alliance." It is an apt title. "Tuberculosis in patients with co-existing HIV infection may develop the disease more rapidly"[28]. However, there is no evidence to suggest that HIV infected individuals with tuberculosis are more infectious than non-HIV infected people.

In countries where there is a high incidence of HIV, the rate of tuberculosis is also high. As the virus weakens the immune system, so TB, the opportunist, is given the chance to take hold. Effectively, the emergence of HIV over the past 20 years has in some parts of the world been the primary driver behind the growing incidence of the disease that we see today.

Summary

Tuberculosis is a bacterial infection that usually attacks the lungs, but can occur in almost any part of the body. It is not a new disease and fortunately, we know quite a lot about it. We are not looking for a cure; we have one! TB is an airborne disease and there is a chance if someone with the disease in their lungs exhales the bacteria that someone else may breathe it in and become infected. Nobody is 'immune' to tuberculosis; everyone is potentially susceptible.

If someone does become infected it does not mean that they will become ill. It must be remembered that latent TB infection is very common. One in three people have come across the bacteria at some point in their lives. However, it is estimated that about 10% of those infected will go on to develop active TB disease at some point in time.

Active TB disease generally develops from latent infection when someone has prolonged and sustained contact with an infectious person. Thereby 'overloading' the immune system to the point where it cannot be contained as a latent infection any more. Active disease might also occur when a person's health is compromised because of social circumstances, poverty, life-style or by another health complication such as HIV. A healthy constitution is probably the best defense against developing active TB disease.

Tuberculosis can become resistant to the drugs used to treat the disease. TB is curable as long as medication is taken correctly and for the right length of time. Some TB patient's non-adherence with medication regimes, is creating a situation where potentially in the future completely incurable strains of the disease could become more prevalent. TB patients have the responsibility to ensure this does not happen by taking their medication properly.

HIV is one of the main reasons why there has been such an increase in incidence of the disease in some parts of the world. Although the two diseases are 'linked' in so much as they seem to 'assist' each other, TB and

HIV are two different diseases. It should be remembered that just because someone has TB, it does not mean that they are HIV-positive. It is just one of many possible factors why someone with latent TB infection may go on to develop active TB disease.

In conclusion, below is a list of some of the more famous public figures from the pages of history that have suffered with tuberculosis. If you have or have had tuberculosis, you are in very good company!

- King Amenophis IV and his wife Nefertiti (1360BC)
- King Louis XIII, King of France (1601-1643)
- Henri Purcell (1658-1695)
- Marquise de Pompadour (1721-1764)
- Nicolo Paganini (1782-1840)
- Carl Maria Von Weber (1786-1826)
- John Keats (1795-1821)
- Napoleon II, King of Rome, Duke of Reichstadt (1811-1832)
- Frederick Chopin (1818-1848)
- Emily Brönte (1818-1848)
- Anne Brönte (1820-1849)
- Edward Grieg (1843-1907)
- Robert Louis Stevenson (1850-1894)
- Anton Chekhov (1860-1904)
- St. Therese of Liseux (1872-1897)
- Igor Stravinsky (1882-1971)
- D.H. Lawrence (1885-1930)
- George Orwell (1903-1950)
- Vivien Leigh (1913-1967)

Chapter 4

HOW IS TUBERCULOSIS DIAGNOSED ?

"Coughs and Sneezes Spread Diseases!"

Anon - Ministry of Health 1942

In Chapter 3 we read that tuberculosis is a disease spread by bacteria when an infected person with active TB disease in their lungs coughs. It can also happen if someone infected with tuberculosis sneezes, shouts or sings (but probably to a lesser degree). Diagnosing latent TB infection and active TB disease is challenging in today's modern world for reasons that will be discussed in this chapter.

Diagnosis of latent TB infection uses methods such as tuberculin skin tests (TST), and more recently, blood tests using entirely new techniques (although not in widespread use at present). Clinicians diagnose active TB disease by normally involving methods such as clinical judgment based on symptoms of active TB disease, chest X-ray, and sputum smear microscopy and growing the bacteria in a culture. There are about 15 new diagnostic tools in the development pipeline at the time of writing [1].

Diagnosis of latent TB infection
The benefits of knowing that someone is latently infected with TB are:

• To know if a person who has been exposed to active TB disease and has been infected (for example in the situation where a contact tracing exercise is being conducted).

- To identify latently infected individuals so that they can be put on preventative TB treatment if it is considered there is a risk of developing active TB disease (for example HIV-positive or otherwise immuno-compromised the elderly and the very young).

- To discover whether someone already has latent TB infection prior to BCG vaccination. If someone already has latent TB infection there is little point in vaccination against the disease, as they have already been exposed. (The BCG vaccination is not practiced in every country of the world and there is some debate about its usefulness. The BCG vaccination is discussed further in chapter 5).

Prior to the BCG vaccination program in the UK and other countries, individuals were screened for TB using the tuberculin skin tests (TST). Increasingly these are becoming of little diagnostic value on their own for several reasons. People who have been vaccinated with the BCG usually give a false positive skin test result. Children, the elderly and the immuno-compromised (such as those with HIV), can give a false positive skin test result because of their impaired immune system. However, these skin tests are in wide usage globally. Therefore, it is useful to review the nature of these tests.

The Heaf test was the preferred method for mass screening in the UK. Tuberculin purified protein derivative (PPD) (a heat treated and 'tamed' form of the tuberculosis bacteria, which is not harmful), is smeared on the skin and small puncture sites are created with a gun apparatus containing six needles. They do not penetrate very far into the skin. It does not hurt and does not usually scar. The test is normally carried out on the inside of the forearm. The test results can then be 'read' with the naked eye after seven days to grade a negative or positive response [2]. Reading Heaf test results is complicated.

The Mantoux test is used in the United States and endorsed by the American Thoracic Society and the CDC. It is very similar in principle, with the exception that a single injection site is made into the skin in the same place as the Heaf test. A stronger strength of tuberculin PPD is used and a lump on the arm is measured after 48-72 hours to identify a positive or negative result [3]. A positive result means that the person has reacted to the tuberculin PPD. It does not necessarily mean that you will become infectious or have active TB disease. It could mean that at some point you breathed in some of the bacteria.

However, your TB specialist may decide to put you on medication as a precaution to stop you from developing TB disease. This is termed 'prophylaxis' i.e., taking medical action or giving treatment to prevent development of disease [4]. (More about preventative treatment is discussed in the next chapter). A negative result would suggest that at the time the test was taken, you did not have latent TB infection or active TB disease. However, this is not conclusive. The test may be falsely negative when using skin tests in a person who has been recently infected. It usually takes two to 10 weeks after being exposed to a person with TB disease for the skin test to show a positive result [5].

The landscape has changed with regard tuberculosis. Essentially, a test that is over 100 years old is being used to identify a disease that is doing very well in a world that has changed a lot in that time and faces new problems. It was Dr Robert Koch's discovery of the tubercle bacillus in the late nineteenth century that led to what he called 'tuberculin' being developed. Essentially derived from heat-treated TB bacteria, it was later developed further by von Pirquet for use as a skin test in 1907 and it is still used today [6].

Each country has its own TB guidelines and there are differences in the approach to control the disease. As mentioned in the US, the Mantoux test is more widely used and endorsed by the CDC (Center for Disease Control) and the American Thoracic Society. In the UK, at the time of writing, the Heaf test is being phased out and the country is becoming more reliant on the Mantoux test, although at present Mantoux is unlicensed for use.

The UK Department of Health was asked whether the government was considering any of the newly available technology, which is more sensitive and reliable than the Heaf and Mantoux test. They replied; "The Department of Health is aware of the need for improved methods for the detection of tuberculosis infection. The matter is currently under consideration by the National Institute for Clinical Excellence (NICE)". At this time, new guidance from NICE had not yet been published.

New technologies that could be considered to replace Heaf and Mantoux are QuantiFERON-TB and T-SPOT.*TB*. The QuantiFERON–TB test (QFT) was approved by the FDA in the US in 2001. It is a blood test that measures a person's immune reaction to *Mycobacterium tuberculosis*; the bacterium that causes TB. QFT works by having a blood sample drawn from the patient, which is mixed with antigens – the protein substances that produce an immune response – and controls. Then the blood is incubated for 16-24 hours.

There are a number of advantages and disadvantages to the QFT test. One advantage is that the test reduces the risk of testing interpretations and bias and one disadvantage is that there is limited knowledge and experience with QFT tuberculosis testing.

One of the best alternative tests for consideration is T-SPOT.*TB*, which is a blood test that works in a completely different way to the old skin tests. There is substantial published evidence that the test is a marked improvement over the existing skin tests [7]. It is an easy and rapid technique to detect latent TB infection in the blood. It provides an accurate result irrespective of previous BCG vaccination. It can also help in the more accurate selection of TB contacts for preventative treatment by eliminating the false positives produced by tuberculin skin testing [8] and T-SPOT.*TB* works well in very vulnerable people such as babies, the elderly and those with weak immune systems. Probably the most useful advance of this new technology is its ability to detect latent TB infection, even in those who are immuno-compromised [9].

Diagnosis of active TB disease

The symptoms of active TB disease were discussed in the previous chapter. If an individual presents to a doctor with these symptoms it will alert him that the patient may have TB. As well as clinical judgement there are several other tests that are used to confirm a doctor's suspicions.

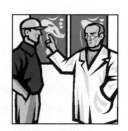

The easiest test is the chest X-ray. Areas in the lungs affected by TB appear as white spots that may be cavities and there may also be some abnormal shadowing. However, the chest X-ray may be misleading as other lung diseases can be confused with TB and it is difficult to distinguish between current TB and previous TB which has been successfully treated. Therefore further investigations may be required [10].

The scientist, Robert Koch's method of staining TB bacteria, which enabled their visualization for the first time, provides the basis for two tests. The first (and quickest) is a 'sputum smear' test. The sample of phlegm is examined under a microscope to see if any TB bacteria show up after it is stained and washed using the technique described in the previous chapter. If the 'sputum smear' is positive for TB, this is termed "smear positive". The result of the test is graded in terms of 'plus's' (+ to +++) indicating low, medium or high amounts of acid-fast bacilli. The higher the result the more infectious the person is likely to be.

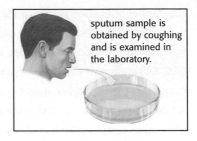

sputum sample is obtained by coughing and is examined in the laboratory.

If you have active TB disease your TB specialist will want a lot of sputum. The specialist can then monitor whether your treatment is working by looking for acid-fast bacilli in the samples that you subsequently provide after treatment is commenced. As the TB bacteria are killed by drugs, you will find that sputum smear results get better. Eventually, the grading of the smear test will indicate that you are no longer infectious. **This will only happen if the medication has been taken according to your doctor's instructions.**

TB is a complex subject. A negative sputum smear test result does not mean that one is cured. It simply means that the person is no longer infectious and no longer actively coughing up TB bacilli. In addition, a TB specialist will want to carry out a second test called 'sputum culture'. This means attempting to grow TB bacilli under laboratory conditions over a period of time; this usually takes about eight to 12 weeks [11].

If either a sputum smear test or sputum culture is positive during TB treatment, it means that TB bacilli are still present and TB treatment needs to continue. Even when you do produce your first negative sputum culture, your TB specialist will want to carry out further test before he is satisfied you are cured and tells you to stop treatment.

Contact Tracing

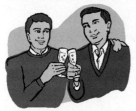

Tuberculosis is a 'notifiable' disease. That means that the authorities will be advised that you have the disease [12] to ensure that diseases can be monitored to see how and if they are present in the population. It is from this information that we are able to create statistics. It is also the way we can prove that TB continues to increase globally in terms of prevalence. Your doctors may need to test people with whom you have been in contact to see if they have also been infected. Usually, this will be confined to close contacts, such as family and people with whom you live or see regularly [13]. You may be asked for a list of their names and other details.

Summary

The diagnosis of tuberculosis, for the most part, relies on a test that is over 100 years old. It is inadequate in diagnosing latent TB infection and some forms of the active disease in the world today. Research and development into new diagnostics for tuberculosis has been neglected over the past few decades since tuberculosis was deemed to have been brought under control and had become treatable in the developed world.

The World Health Organization recognizes the need for research and development into new diagnostic tools as do other major organizations. There also already exits new technology such as T-SPOT.*TB* that are far more sensitive and reliable in those who might produce a false positive result to the skin test. It is important that tests such as these are rapidly introduced.

Chapter 5

TREATMENT AND ADHERENCE

"Venienti occurite morbo - Confront disease at its onset"

Persius (Antus Persius Flaccus) AD 34-62

Tuberculosis treatment falls into two categories: *preventative*, which means trying to stop people from getting TB in the first place, and *remedial*: treating the disease when it occurs [1].

TB Treatment: Preventative

The three most important preventative measures for tuberculosis involve the BCG vaccination, maintaining a healthy lifestyle and pre-emptive treatment for TB if found to be latently infected.

BCG vaccination (Bacille Calmette-Guerin)

In the United Kingdom, the BCG vaccine used to be given at school between the ages of 10-14, a few weeks after a Heaf test. It usually leaves a small scar and is given in the left-upper arm. The future of the BCG vaccination program in the UK is in a state of flux at the time of writing. However, where there is a high incidence of TB, for example in inner city areas, some TB specialists prefer to give the BCG vaccination at a very young age, often as young as only a few weeks old. Its safety is undisputed: the effectiveness of the vaccine itself is, however, a contentious issue. BCG vaccination programs will depend on local and regional TB control policy.

In some US states, vaccination with BCG is not a routine undertaking, as its usefulness is felt to be uncertain. Additionally, because the BCG vaccine contains 'tamed' and safe bacteria, when a vaccinated person has a Heaf or Mantoux test after vaccination they often produce a positive result [2]. It is believed that this impairs the usefulness of later Heaf testing.

When asked about the different attitudes of the UK and USA towards the BCG vaccination, Senior Medical Officer, Dr Jane Leese from the Communicable Diseases branch of the UK Department of Health said: "The Americans are not convinced of the benefits of BCG and believe it interferes with the tuberculin skin test as a diagnostic aid, and it is true that most people will develop a low-grade positive skin test response after BCG. In the UK, we do not find this a problem. It is also true that trials of BCG have shown widely differing effectiveness - in general, the nearer the tropics, the less effective it seems to be and the reason for the variation is not understood."

The BCG vaccination remains an area of debate in terms of its effectiveness because many people that are vaccinated still contract the disease. A mass vaccination program can also have another adverse effect: people may fail to recognize that TB causes their symptoms because they have been vaccinated against it, and assume they are immune. Complacency over the disease has been blamed as one of the factors for the rise in the incidence of TB, especially in the developed world [3].

The first recombined tuberculosis vaccine entered clinical trials in the United States in 2004 sponsored by the National Institute of Allergy and Infectious Diseases (NIAID). It was recently reported that a DNA TB vaccine given with conventional chemotherapy can accelerate the disappearance of bacteria as well as protecting against re-infection in mice but it may take four to five years to be available in humans.

A healthy lifestyle – the best defense against developing TB disease
In chapter three, we learned that if someone has latent TB infection, the immune system keeps the TB bacteria 'in-check'. We know that there are circumstances that can have an impact on health such as poverty, malnutrition, and poor living conditions all leading to health inequalities. Our social circumstances and lifestyle have an impact on our health and wellbeing. When the immune system is compromised, its ability to keep TB bacteria 'in-check' is impaired. This can lead to latent TB infection becoming active TB disease.

The best defense against developing active TB disease is to have as healthy lifestyle as possible. Basically, this means eating healthily, drinking alcohol in moderation, not smoking, and not using illegal substances. As a rule of thumb, active TB disease generally occurs when something else causes us to have poor health.

The same is true of other health complications, such as HIV, that are unidentified or untreated. If someone knows they are HIV positive they have the choice of taking anti-retroviral therapy (the drugs used to manage HIV). These drugs reduce the amount of virus in the body by preventing its replication. As a consequence, the immune system if damaged, has a chance to recover to a degree. If the immune system is functioning as well as it can, the risk of developing active TB disease from latent TB is reduced.

This could be considered as one good reason to be tested for HIV, if you think you may have been at risk of contracting the virus. There is a benefit to knowing if you are HIV-positive because more people with HIV develop active TB disease than any other opportunistic infection.

Pre-emptive treatment – Chemoprophylaxis

Chemoprophylaxis is the use of a chemical agent to prevent the development of a disease. Medication can be taken pre-emptively to prevent active TB disease from occurring in the first place. However, there are challenges around identifying latent TB infection in the world we live in today. These were discussed in the previous chapter. For preventative treatment to be successful, we need to know:

A) Has someone been exposed to an identified case of active TB disease? Are they at risk of developing active TB disease as a consequence?

B) Is there reliable test evidence to conclude that someone has become latently infected with TB?

When tuberculin skin testing (TST) is so unreliable in those who are infants, elderly, malnourished, immuno-compromised, or HIV-positive, clearly there is a need for a more definitive test[4].

For the most part, the decision to prescribe pre-emptive TB treatment is based on clinical judgment as to whether an infected individual is at risk of developing active TB disease.

TB Treatment: Remedial

If you are diagnosed with active TB disease, your doctor will want to put you on the right medication to treat it. There are a variety of drugs worldwide that are used in combination with other drugs. If you have fully drug-sensitive tuberculosis, you will usually be given a combination of the following:

- **Isoniazid (INH):** An inexpensive and highly effective drug, which will always be given if you have drug-sensitive tuberculosis, unless there are specific reasons for not giving it to you. Its only common side effect is peripheral neuropathy (tingling and numbness in your fingers, hands, toes or feet, which can sometimes be quite painful). This is more likely to happen if you have diabetes or a problem with alcohol or kidneys, or if you have HIV. High doses of Pyridoxine (Vitamin B6) can sometimes help in these cases.

To ensure that hepatitis, which is a rarer side effect, does not occur, your TB specialist will perform special blood tests. Mental health problems are even rarer. Most people tolerate this drug rather well and it is very effective. Isoniazid is given in combination with rifampicin.

- **Rifampicin (RIF):** Like isoniazid, this drug is a key component of the anti-tuberculosis regime. It will always be included unless there is a good reason not to. Occasionally, the liver has problems coping with this drug, and you are more likely to suffer from this if you have previously had liver disease. As with isoniazid, your doctor will want to take blood tests to ensure you are tolerating the drug.

Rifampicin can cause other minor side effects. For example, it might stain the urine, tears, saliva or sperm an orange color. This may seem odd at first but it is not something about which you need to be alarmed. Note also that you should not wear soft contact lenses as they may stain orange and it might also make you more sensitive to the sun so ensure you use a sun block.

Female patients may find that Rifampicin has the effect of making the contraceptive pill and implants less effective. Women should talk to their doctors about alternative birth control measures.

Anyone taking methadone for drug dependency may require an adjustment in the methadone dosage. Rifampicin can change the way methadone is absorbed; therefore, withdrawal symptoms may be noted and the dose will need to be re-assessed.

- **Ethambutol (EMB):** This drug is normally prescribed for two months initial treatment if the patient is unable to take Isoniazid. (Incidentally, isoniazid resistance is the most common; this is not surprising as it is one of the most commonly prescribed anti-tuberculosis drugs.) Side effects of ethambutol are largely confined to visual disturbance; color blindness and restriction of the field of vision are common when excessive doses have been taken, or if the person taking the drug has kidney problems. For this reason, it is not used for the treatment of young children.

  The TB specialist will carry out tests for color blindness, much like the ones that you had at school. A number made up of dots, hidden among dots of appropriately contrasting colours. This is called the Ishihara test. Ethambutol dosage is prescribed according to weight. The doctor may adjust the dose or change the drug completely if visual problems occur.

- **Pyrazinamide (PZA):** This drug is useful in the treatment of tuberculosis meningitis because it penetrates into the brain substance. There is a barrier around the brain which many drugs find hard to pass through. Liver problems may also occasionally occur with this drug.

- **Streptomycin (SM):** This drug is administered as an intra-muscular injection in the muscle of the buttock. Once again, the clinician will take blood samples to see how the liver and kidneys are coping with the drug. People who have had liver or kidney problems in the past are more at risk of developing serious side effects. Other side effects include numbness and tingling in and around your mouth, and long-term usage can cause permanent damage to your hearing. It is really important to tell your doctor if you experience ringing in the ears (tinnitus). In the UK, this drug is rarely used now with the exception of resistant types of tuberculosis.

Treatment of Multidrug-resistant tuberculosis
The patient who does not respond to isoniazid and rifampicin, is considered to have Multidrug-resistant tuberculosis (MDR-TB). This is more serious, as it may take longer to treat. MDR-TB is treated with what are called 'second-line' drugs. The side effects with these agents may be more severe than with the above listed drugs and second-line drugs are only used if necessary.

Although, MDR-TB is still relatively uncommon in the US and UK, it is growing in incidence globally. The World Health Organization believe that the incidence of MDR-TB may actually be three times higher than its recorded incidence and could exceed one million [5]. MDR-TB is not a major problem in countries implementing tuberculosis control over a period of several years and in accordance with their national guidelines. Botswana, Chile, Cuba, the Czech Republic, and Uruguay have all showed very low prevalence of MDR-TB, confirming that efficient tuberculosis control prevents the outset and spread of MDR-TB throughout the years [6]. The same can be said for developed countries with long histories of TB control, such as Australia, Canada, Denmark, France, and The Netherlands. Data taken from the US and UK suggest that MDR-TB is not a major public health issue; it is confined to specific groups, including immigrants, refugees and the homeless [7].

The WHO recommended strategy to control tuberculosis is recognized as the best method of TB control. It prevents drug-resistance and ensures continuity and adherence of patients to TB treatment. However, MDR-TB threatens the strategy to control TB. This is because the strategy relies on first-line drugs used in standardized short-course treatment. These drugs are ineffective against MDR-TB. Consequently, the number of patients with MDR-TB is growing. This is a significant infectious pool for the proliferation of new MDR-TB cases [8]. Therefore, second-line TB treatment will be required to successfully treat and cure the disease.

Generally, drugs used to treat MDR-TB are outside the budgets of the most resource-limited countries of the world where 80% of TB occurs. In the past, this problem had even led some to say that MDR-TB in some settings may be untreatable [9]. Thankfully, this is no longer the case. In response, the World Health Organization created a working group to address the problem. Soon after the creation of this working group in 2000, a sub-group was formed called the Green Light Committee (GLC). Its ultimate aim was to increase access to second-line anti-tuberculosis drugs needed to treat MDR-TB in a rational way. As a pilot project it was called DOTS-Plus. Today, it is no longer a pilot and fully integrated into the Stop TB strategy.

The mechanism works as follows: the working group negotiated a substantial reduction in the prices of second-line drugs with the pharmaceutical industry, thereby achieving a major cost reduction. Countries that have sound TB control programs in place can apply to the GLC for access to these much less expensive second-line drugs. The GLC assess the TB control program for suitability. It is important that second-line drugs are used rationally because misuse could lead to further drug-resistance and there are NO third-line drugs for treating TB.

Applications to the GLC must also verify that treatment of MDR-TB is provided free of charge to the patients [10]. It is now possible and cost effective to address all forms of TB. Even in the most resource-limited countries of the world there is the chance of a cure for all. It is important that this program to address MDR-TB is rapidly scaled up.

Being treated for MDR-TB is not easy. There are often a lot of tablets to take and the side effects of being treated with second-line drugs are harder to tolerate. Your doctor will be able to tell you about the side effects you may get if you require treatment with second-line drugs. You will also be closely monitored on this type of medication. Some of the side effects of TB treatment are minor while others can be more serious. If you are having any side effects, tell your TB specialist or nurse about them.

The side effects listed below are, according to the USA's Center for Disease Prevention and Control's Questions and Answers about TB [5], are more serious and you should contact your TB specialist or nurse immediately if you experience them.

- No appetite
- Nausea
- Vomiting
- Fever for three days or more
- Abdominal pain
- Tingling in the fingers or toes
- Skin rash
- Easy bruising or bleeding
- Aching joints
- Dizziness
- Tingling or numbness around the mouth
- Blurred or altered vision
- Ringing in the ears
- Hearing loss

How long will I be on treatment?
When people have healthy immune systems and drug-sensitive TB, treatment will usually last for six to nine months. However, it can be longer, possibly as long as two years [6]. Treatment for people who are immuno-compromised,

with HIV for example, may take longer, and it could, actually last years. Clearly, therefore, a healthy immune system assists in combating the disease.

Taking your medication

If you have TB disease and start treatment you are likely to feel better within several weeks. It is also likely that you will be non-infectious after this period of time [7]. The doctor will be able to tell you whether you are infectious or not from your sputum samples.

Even if you feel better and the doctor says you are not infectious, this does not mean that you are cured. TB bacilli take a long time to kill because they replicate so slowly. They may be hiding somewhere but the doctor will know from the sputum culture samples. All of the bacteria must be killed or the TB disease may come back. Some people make the mistake of stopping the medication when they feel better. This can lead to treatment failure [8].

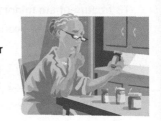

NB: *You will find a TB Treatment Chart in Appendix B to help you take your TB medication*

Treatment Failure

Rosy Weston, a Senior GUM/HIV pharmacist at St Mary's Hospital London, has had experience with problems that can lead to treatment failure. She says: "There are two main reasons why individuals may not adhere to medication. First, there is 'intentional non-adherence'. This occurs when the individual makes a decision to miss a dose or change the way the medication is taken. An example of this is when you know that a certain drug makes you feel really sick just after taking the medicine so you decide - or take advice from someone - not to take the drug.

"Another example, which is very common, involves taking a course of antibiotics. Although you have been recommended to take the drugs for ten days, for example, you feel so well after five days that you stop.

"Then there is unintentional non-adherence. This occurs simply when an individual is unaware that they may be taking the drugs incorrectly e.g. the wrong dose or simply forgetting to take a dose."

There is an element of truth in Francis Bacon's comment that: "The remedy is worse than the disease"[15]. Like many forms of chemotherapy, TB treatment can have unpleasant side effects that are difficult on individuals. (The second-line drugs used in the treatment of Multidrug-resistant tuberculosis are particularly challenging). In some ways, the side effects can feel worse than the disease itself, and avoiding unpleasant side effects may be the object of stopping medication. It is extremely important to continue with the medication. If problems with side effects arise, consult with both the TB specialist or pharmacist about them to ensure that you are doing all that can be done to overcome them.

Prior to beginning a TB medication regime, it may be worthwhile to ask the doctor, nurse or pharmacist the following questions:

• What are the most common side effects and what should I look for?
• How soon after taking the drugs can they appear and how long do they last?
• What can I do to reduce the symptoms or are there any other drugs I can take to help?
• Are there any information leaflets I should read?

Poor adherence is the main reason for relapse into active TB disease [16]. The doctor can test the blood and urine, make random pill counts and check prescriptions. The clinician will know if you are not taking your pills! In extreme circumstances, you should be aware that if you fail to adhere to treatment and pose a risk to others, you could be incarcerated in the interests of wider public health. You can be responsible for your own health and the health of others and at the same time maintain your civil liberties. It should be noted that different countries have different guidance for dealing with the situation of non-adherence to treatment.

DOT – Directly Observed Therapy

The good news is that if detected and treated properly under medical supervision, most patients with TB recover. Failure to respond to treatment - usually around 5% of cases - occurs in those people who poorly adhere [17]. It can be difficult to take what seems to be a lot of pills for such a long time. There are ways, however, of ensuring adherence and although treatment does take some time, discipline is an essential ingredient in defeating the disease.

Part of the World Health Organization's recommended strategy to control TB is called 'DOT', Directly Observed Therapy. In effect, DOT means that a health care worker or other trusted person is available to help the patient through the TB treatment journey to ensure that treatment is administered effectively through observation [18].

DOT can sometimes feel intrusive but it has major benefits. Not only does the patient always take the pills correctly, but a relationship can build with the person administering DOT. The patient is able to speak with them about side effects as they occur, any fears they may have about the disease and any other problems being encountered.

Summary

As reinforced throughout this book, tuberculosis is a curable disease when treatment is correctly adhered to and only stopped when told to do so by a TB specialist.

TB treatment falls into two categories: Preventative and Remedial. There are challenges in diagnosing latent TB infection in today's world (as discussed in Chapter 4). This impacts the ability to instigate preventative treatment in those who are most vulnerable. For patients with active disease, a minimum of six months is a long time to take medication. There may well be side effects, especially with second-line treatments. It may feel that the TB specialist at times does not understand this.

When patients get to the point that they feel better, are experiencing side effects or possibly have other socio-economic and personal problems, this is the time when they may not adhere to TB treatment or possibly completely stop. This has the potential to lead to drug-resistant strains. Those who develop Multidrug-resistant tuberculosis will be more difficult to treat. Treatment failure is serious. People with TB that are infectious present a risk to public health.

The World Health Organization (WHO) strategy to control TB includes a component called DOT (Directly Observed Therapy). This is when a patient is observed taking their medication. It may happen on every dose of the regimen or occasionally, such as three times a week.

Being on DOT and observed taking your medication can feel intrusive but many people have been cured using this strategy. If you are taking TB medication without support and are finding it difficult, tell your TB specialist. It is likely he or she will be able assign someone to you to administer DOT.

Remember: if someone becomes very ill with TB, is having problems taking their medication and is at risk of developing MDR-TB, or already has a drug-resistant strain, it is possible they will be isolated to ensure successful treatment and also ensure it is not transmitted to anyone else.

Non-adherence to treatment is, in part, causing an increased incidence of MDR-TB. It is threatening the global strategy, DOTS, to control TB. This is because the strategy uses what is called standardized short-course treatment, which means that the drugs used are to treat drug-sensitive strains of TB. If strains become resistant, then standardized short-course treatment will not be effective. In recognition of this, DOTS has evolved to include DOTS-Plus. It is a mechanism whereby second-line drugs used to treat MDR-TB, which are expensive at market prices, can be procured at vastly discounted prices.

Countries that previously could not afford to buy drugs to treat MDR-TB are now in a position to obtain them. Countries must demonstrate that there is a sound DOTS program in place to ensure rational use of second-line drugs and therefore prevent further resistance to second-line drugs.

Chapter 6

UNDERSTANDING ISOLATION

"Isolation is aloneness that feels forced upon you, like a punishment. Solitude is aloneness you choose and embrace. Great things can come out of solitude, out of going to a place where all is quiet except for the beating of your heart".

Jeanne Marie Laskas, Writer, The Washington Post

Isolation as an infection control measure

Isolation is not an experience everyone with TB will go through. For those that do, it can be a difficult and emotional time. TB is a social disease. When someone is found to be infectious with TB, they may need to be isolated to receive treatment and prevent further transmission of infection. Generally, after a few of weeks of treatment, a patient should no longer be infectious [1]. This does not mean that one is cured and full treatment will take longer.

For some cases of TB, isolation is considered an effective method of infection control. This contrasts with old treatment methods when consumptives were sent to TB sanatoriums. People lived together - sometimes for years - in well-ventilated rooms. Sometimes TB sanatoriums were in beautiful surroundings in the mountains or by the side of a lake [2]. Plenty of fresh air was the order of the day. On appearance, it was more like a holiday than a stay in a hospital. Times have changed, however, and instead of living in this type of community, 'isolation' now means just that.

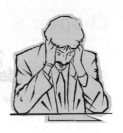

Hospital Isolation

Many people who have been through the hospital isolation experience say that it is the hardest part of having TB. Isolation is in either a negative-pressure room or a room with a closed door, away from other patients. The safest form of isolation is the former. A negative-pressure room is a room where the air pressure is lower than outside the door.

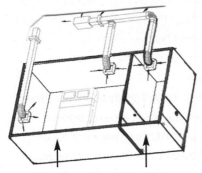

Isolation Room   Ante Room

This means that air can only blow in and not out. If your hospital is very modern, you may not even be aware that there is a mechanism creating this lowered air pressure effect. The mechanism is usually set in an outer wall.

If your room is a negative-pressure room and the weather is very warm, you will not be able to have a fan. The air pressure in the room could be affected and blow infectious TB bacteria under the door. The air pressure does not feel any lower than outside the room. The air also does not seem 'thin' like some people might imagine and in fact, you do not notice a difference at all. As a standard, negative-pressure rooms have two doors. Beyond the door to the room itself there is usually another smaller room or chamber, and a door to the area outside. The isolation room is relatively normal by hospital standards. More often than not there will be a bathroom or shower but the window cannot be opened, as it will affect the negative air pressure.

The wearing of masks by visitors is compulsory and the masks are a special type. The perforations are smaller than those found in standard surgical masks. If the holes are smaller there is less chance of breathing in any TB bacilli.

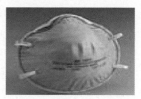

Sample of a mask approved to meet OSHA requirements and CDC guidelines for TB exposure control.

Isolation does not mean being entirely cut off from people. In many cases, you will be allowed to have visitors and the hospital will keep a record of their names. They will be told that by coming into the room they are putting themselves at risk, and are left to make the decision for themselves. A record of their names is kept so that if any of them become infected, effective contact tracing can be carried out.

Visitors may also be required to have a test for TB, give sputum samples or have chest X-rays to ensure they have not contracted the disease. It is unwise to have pregnant women, children, immuno-compromised, or elderly people come to visit you. If these people really want to visit they should be clearly informed of the risks.

How long might I be in isolation?

For some people, the TB experience is worsened not by the disease itself, but the hardships and loneliness of isolation. Isolation may last a long time. Those who have drug-sensitive tuberculosis may only require isolation for two weeks. Others with Multidrug-resistant tuberculosis may require longer, because the drugs used to treat the disease work slower than first-line treatments.

If you have drug-sensitive TB and are adherent with your medication, the doctor should be able to give you a fairly good estimate of your stay. It does help to know how long you are going to be isolated because if you can see the days, and count them down, it seems to make the whole experience easier. Eventually, you will see light at the end of the tunnel. For those who are immuno-compromised or have Multidrug-resistant tuberculosis, the stay will probably be longer. It might also be harder for your doctor to give you an idea when you may be discharged.

Most doctors, particularly in areas where there is a high incidence of the disease, can be quite precise about length of stay. However, there are regional variations in discharge policy and as a result your discharge might be delayed.

Psychological effects of isolation

Isolation brings a unique set of 'coping' problems with it. There is little written about the subject in relation to tuberculosis and the psychological effects. However, there is a study of people placed in isolation following a bone marrow transplant [3]. Isolation is necessary while the transplant is 'taking'; during this time the patients are at risk from a variety of infections. This is because their immune system is artificially suppressed to prevent rejection of the transplant. It is interesting to note that patients are isolated to prevent them from being infected rather than infecting others.

After reviewing a 14-30 day period in isolation [4], the study found that patients suffered depression, anxiety, and disorientation. In addition, some patients complained of concentration difficulties. They also experienced odd sleeping patterns and a feeling of loss of control, which could cause mood swings [5].

There are many similarities between both experiences of isolation. The major difference between the two is that bone marrow transplants are planned, and individuals have some time to prepare themselves mentally prior to the procedure. Having TB is not a planned experience, and the individual is seldom prepared for what follows.

The study further states that: "Patient's concerns are health, family, marital attitudes, financial worries, sexual and social activities, job and daily life, self-image as well as the concerns about the disease itself "[6]. Patients describe the experience as being in a state of limbo or going 'stir crazy'. The report recommends that patients make structures for themselves in 15 minute blocks of time, requiring them to do their own bathing, and formally schedule a time for watching television, making phone calls, exercising and resting. The authors encourage patients to bring in furniture, computers and other items from home, that might increase their comfort and help to occupy and structure their days.

Isolation and your diet
Spending time away from foods that you normally cook and eat can be difficult. Hospital food is well balanced and planned by dieticians. Jane Rowntree, a senior dietician at St. Mary's Hospital in London, understands the difficulties; "Some people have food brought in for them. If they do, then it might help to speak to a dietician. The majority of people who have food brought in for them end up with chocolates and that sort of thing which are not the ideal thing that everybody needs at this time. The thing to do is work out what you want from the hospital menu and what foods you want brought in to you. By eating both, you should get the full spectrum of nutrients you need.

The balance is important because TB, like many illnesses can cause weight loss and a loss of appetite. Athletes have extremely healthy diets and extremely healthy appetites: they eat lots of high carbohydrate foods like bananas, rice, pastas, but these are not very energy dense. Choice of diet is clearly linked with your appetite, and what you can manage at the time. If you have a very good appetite, then that is great. You can eat those sorts of foods, including fruit and vegetables as well. If your appetite is very poor, then obviously you do not want to go for these foods alone because you do not get enough energy from them. You may have to add in some of the things that would not usually be considered particularly healthy; fatty foods for instance.

If your appetite is very poor, it is still possible to obtain the nutrients you need from nutritional supplements. The types of supplements on offer vary and some of them are called 'complete'. This means that one can actually get all nutrients from the supplements. Others are more specific, and are given in relation to the problems being experienced with food. Some of them are designed just to give carbohydrates, some to increase body mass, and others to provide vitamins and minerals. These have a vital role in providing us with the nutrients we need to aid our recovery. If you are having problems with your food, ask to see a dietician."

Isolation and exercise

Isolation rooms are often very small. However, if you feel well enough you should try to do some exercise. You can do this, even if your room is not big enough for exercise equipment. Ask to 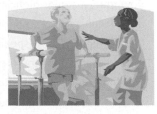 see a physiotherapist who will be able to discuss a suitable program with you. It is helpful to exercise while in isolation to keep muscle tone. If you are not moving around very much, muscle tone can decline rapidly. Psychologically, exercising will help you to feel that you are doing something to help yourself, particularly when it seems that you have lost control over your life. Just as dietary choices help, this also returns a degree of control. When you have TB, there is no better feeling than realizing that you are putting on weight. If you are taking your medication, you must be getting better. It is a bonus if you are getting fit as well.

Isolation in the community
Simply put, isolation in the community means only having transient contact with other people. As mentioned above, the patient should avoid contact with pregnant women, children, the elderly, or anyone who may be immuno-compromised.

This can be difficult if you rely on support services such as day centers: you may not be able to make use of these. You may also be advised not to use public transport, bars, clubs, or restaurants for a while. This can be hard, but it is a necessary precaution. This form of isolation in the community is only temporary. If you take your medication as prescribed then you will eventually be able to lead a normal life again.

Post isolation emotions
You may have to deal with psychological issues after an isolation experience. There is no doubt that a period of isolation does affect people, sometimes in very subtle ways. Even crossing the road can be difficult. When your senses have been deprived in a small space where nothing moves, fast moving cars and buses can be very daunting. Initially, try to generally slow down until you find it possible to return to your normal lifestyle. This is particularly important with any potentially hazardous activity such as driving, operating machinery, cooking, and other tasks. Take your time and concentrate.

After leaving isolation, you may awake to be totally disorientated by your 'new' surroundings, especially on the first few nights at home. You may also find that you dream about being in the isolation room, or have nightmares.

This is a natural way for your mind to heal after a bad experience. If you are upset, talk to someone about your difficulties. If you have an established relationship with a psychologist, psychiatrist or counselor, it is likely that you will probably see them again after discharge. Ask to see them if you do not already have a regular appointment. Talk about how you are acclimatizing to your new freedom, about sleep patterns, side effects, and any other concerns 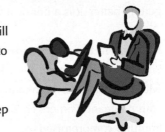 you may have. One of the benefits of being on the DOT program is that you will be building a relationship with someone that has been assigned to your case. It is likely they will be able to offer you the benefit of their experience with regard to the problems discussed.

It is common to fear that the disease will return. Like everyone else, you may get a cold from time to time. Do not immediately jump to the conclusion that it is TB; this is easily done. Be aware of your own body and if you are concerned, give your doctor a sputum sample, and he will be able to tell you how you are doing, and allay your fears.

Look to your future, and make plans. TB, like many bad experiences, can be turned into a positive life changing experience. Eventually, the restrictions on your freedom will be lifted and the DOT and medication will stop. You will still need regular check-ups, and your doctor may carry out the occasional chest X-ray to ensure all is well.

Summary

Not everybody is placed in isolation but for those that are it can be the worst aspect of having the disease. Try to structure your time and do not vegetate if you are well enough to be as active as you can be in one room.

Bring some personal belongings to the room for extra comfort. Change the room around because it will make you feel useful to have some control over the environment. Make sure that people respect your privacy and knock before they enter. Try and do some exercise, as there is likely to be some muscle wasting if you are ill and inactive. You do not need any special equipment to do sit-ups or press ups if you feel well enough. The best part of the TB treatment is that you start to feel better very quickly. You could also ask to speak to a physiotherapist for further advice.

If it is possible, it would be helpful for your TB specialist to give you an idea of when you might be discharged from isolation. If you have an idea of when you might be discharged it will make a big difference to your attitude. If you are unfortunate and do not get a clear answer from your TB specialist, do not panic. Most people do leave isolation eventually.

Keeping a journal could be very useful. It is worth noting that there are many famous writers in the past who have had TB. Have you always wanted to write a book? If you are in isolation, it could be a good time to write it! It is a wonderful feeling to finally walk out of isolation and into the world again. However, you may find that there are restrictions to your freedom with regard to social contact. Also, you will have to continue to take your medication correctly.

When the TB specialist discharges you, he or she will feel that you pose a minimal infection risk. This would have been established following several negative sputum smear results. Other criteria for discharge include absence of fever for at least a week and a good degree of weight gain.

You may be asked when you leave the isolation in the hospital to abide by some simple rules, in effect, isolation in the community. This means having social contact for only limited periods of time. You will probably be required to attend the chest clinic at least once a month. It is possible that your TB specialist might ask that you be assisted in taking your medication (see Directly Observed Therapy in Chapter 5). He will also want more sputum samples so that he can check that you remain sputum smear negative, and continue to monitor the results of sputum smear and culture samples.

If you become sputum smear positive again, your doctor is likely to re-admit you. This will happen if the medication is not working. However, it should not happen if you are taking the medication correctly. Do not assume that you have been discharged because you are cured. TB treatment takes time. If you are having trouble taking medication on your own, tell your TB specialist. It is likely that he will be able to engage a TB nurse to assist you in your treatment.

Chapter 7

LIFESTYLE MANAGEMENT

"Life isn't finished for us yet! We're going to live."

Anton Chekov

The TB treatment journey is a long one and it is not only about taking pills. Although taking your medication is the first priority, there are other things that you can do to help you get better and prevent relapse. Many people start to think about their lifestyle during and after a long illness and try to make improvements.

We have established in this book that an individual with active TB disease, if they have TB in the lungs, is likely to be non-infectious after about two to three weeks of TB treatment. If you were suffering fatigue as you became ill, you will probably, with treatment, have a lot more energy than you did before. The journey is not over yet and some people make the mistake of stopping medication only to become ill again. There is at least six months of pill taking ahead at this stage. While you are on TB treatment, there are other things you might want to consider that will aid your recovery.

Formulate a plan that encompasses the following elements:

- Eating a healthy diet
- Getting plenty of rest and sleep
- Taking up some exercise
- Dealing with psychological issues (if there are any)

You may not wish to do all of the above but you can you take what you want from these and leave the rest. Although there is a lot that you can do to help yourself, these points above are meant as suggestions for your consideration.

Eating a healthy diet

It is possible that you have lost some weight, perhaps quite a lot, while you have been ill with tuberculosis. You will find that when the medication starts to work, you may feel hungrier. This is a very good sign. It is beneficial to the patient's psychological wellbeing to see that he or she is putting on weight. It means that you are getting better.

A healthy lifestyle with healthy eating habits is important for everyone. It can also be considered as a preventative measure to prevent latent TB infection from becoming active TB disease, and prevents many other problems. After a period of illness, it is important to eat the right foods to aid convalescence.

Nutrition plays a key role in maintaining a healthy lifestyle. According to Jane Rowntree, "It is a very important issue; the body needs different sorts of nutrients to function effectively. A lot of people only look at their weight as a measure of how good their diet is.

People may overeat and be overweight, but if they do not eat the right foods they can still be deficient in vitamins and minerals. The overall picture of what people are eating is important. It is well known that poor nutrition can affect the immune system."

Eating meat and fish may be important in the treatment and prevention of TB. Recently, a study of Asian immigrants in south London found that vegetarians who ate no fish, meat or dairy products, were at least eight times more likely to develop TB than those who ate meat or dairy products every day [1].

The outcome suggests that a deficiency of vitamin B12 (provided almost entirely by foods from animal sources or fortified foods) increases the risk 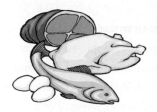 of developing TB. Appropriate intake is necessary to keep your immune system as strong as possible. A lack of vitamin D can also affect the strength of your immune response. There are some interesting studies going on at the time of writing that are looking into the benefits of vitamin D supplements to help prevent latent TB infection becoming active TB disease – the results are not available yet.

Jane Rowntree says; "There are sometimes problems getting all of the nutrients you need. Vitamin B12 is concentrated in a lot of animal foods, such as milk, eggs and cheese. If you are a vegetarian or a vegan there may be a problem. It is important to make sure that you are getting enough before you develop any deficiency symptoms. If you do not eat meat, fish or dairy products you can, for example, increase your intake of yeast extracts. These contain a high concentration of vitamin B12 and contain no animal by-products. "High levels of vitamin B12 are found in some breakfast cereals. A lot of them are fortified with vitamins and minerals in any case. Regular consumption will ensure adequate vitamin intake."

If your medication includes isoniazid or cycloserine (a drug used in the treatment of MDR-TB), you will be given a vitamin B6 (pyridoxine) supplement to counter some of the side effects. Certain nuts are good sources of B6, but it would be difficult to get a large enough dose of vitamin B6 from food alone. Your doctor will ensure you get the correct dosage. A simple solution would be to take a multivitamin once daily. This will provide you with the recommended daily amount of what your body needs. It is important to note, however, that if you are planning any major dietary changes it is wise to consult a dietician. Your doctor will be able to refer you to one.

Getting plenty of rest and sleep

In the days when people went to a TB sanatorium to convalesce, rest was considered one of the most important factors in getting people well again. Indeed, before the days of TB medication some people with good food and rest did recover from the disease. There is a wonderfully funny book that was written in the 1940s by a woman who documented her experience of a one-year stay at a TB sanatorium. Her name was Betty Macdonald and the book was titled *"The Plague and I"*. Particularly funny are her descriptions of staff who were looking after her and how getting out of bed was absolutely forbidden! On a few occasions she was caught wandering around by the nursing staff and she would be reprimanded.

While you are ill with active TB disease you may not feel like getting out of bed but as you get better, you may feel like doing more. Activities should all be done in moderation to avoid over exhaustion. Pushing yourself too hard could set you back because your body needs time to repair itself. Good food and bed rest are important components for recovering from active TB disease. Rest is not necessarily sleep, rest means allowing yourself to be comfortable and do very little. Sleep is the time when our bodies repair themselves.

If you cannot sleep, tell your TB specialist who will be able to prescribe something to help you sleep. Allow your body to get as much sleep as it needs without having to be shocked awake by an alarm clock. Get at least the recommended minimum of eight hours, if not more. Sometimes, you may feel a little guilty for taking so much rest and sleeping late but remember that you have been very ill. Rest and sleep are an important part of recovering from any illness.

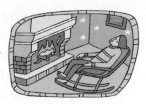

Taking up some exercise

As previously mentioned, everything you do should be in moderation. In time, you will need less rest and your body performance should be moving toward getting back to normal. If you have been isolated and started an exercise regime, try to keep it up once you have been discharged. If you were not isolated, why not start a gentle exercise regimen when you feel able?

Do not do more than you feel capable of doing. A brisk half hour walk is good for your heart and lungs; if you can do more, it would be beneficial. However, do not over exert yourself. You may also want to consider doing some exercise that tones and strengthens your muscles. If you have been isolated you will not have had much room to move around and a brisk walk would have been out of the question. Also, if you had been confined to bed at home you may have experienced some muscle wasting.

There is no need for an expensive gym membership because quite a lot can be done with no equipment at all. Try some gentle stretching exercises; perhaps progress to some press-ups or sit-ups. Remind your body what it is there to do: it is the vehicle in which you travel around! If you have not exercised much in the past, perhaps now is a good time to start.

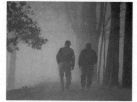

You may have also lost some unwanted weight while having TB. Ask a doctor or dietician what your optimum weight should be and remember that now is not the time for a weight loss diet. With healthy eating.habits and exercise you may find, that you look and feel better after six months of TB treatment than you did before you first became ill. Having a disease can focus attention on our health in a positive way, making all the difference to our future health prospects. It is also helpful in maintaining self-esteem.

Dealing with psychological issues
Having tuberculosis can have more effect on you than just a physical impact. Many people experience feelings of guilt and/or anger at being infected, feeling dirty and damage to self-esteem. Your perception of your own body image also may be affected because of weight loss and other symptoms of the disease.

There is often 'stigma' (shame, embarrassment, humiliation) attached to having any infectious disease and tuberculosis is no different. Much of this is due to historical perceptions of tuberculosis. The reality is that TB is just another infection. You may have feelings of guilt and might also be wondering or know that you have infected someone else. We can transmit the disease to one another and this is not the fault of anyone if they did not know that they had TB in the first place.

Stigma may come from several directions: the feelings of other patients, healthcare workers and even health facilities. Stigma associated with TB appears to be universal. Persons have been known to hesitate or choose not to disclose their TB status to family, friends, and co-workers out of fear of being socially ostracized, in addition to losing their employment.

In some cases, personal rejection occurs as a result of the stigma surrounding TB. Stigma has been shown to hinder adherence to treatment and therefore, there is a need for effective strategies to alleviate it.

Nurses that interact with patients and help to deliver healthcare services can particularly play a key role in helping to lift the barrier of stigma. Their understanding of the disease and subsequent attitudes and perceptions can strongly influence the community in which the patient is living. This is particularly relevant in geographical areas where nurses are sometimes the only health provider in rural suroundings or resource-limited countries fighting to stave off TB and MDR-TB.

Anger is a common reaction to discovering you have TB. You may wonder who gave it to you but there is little point in worrying with questions. You can become stressed trying to answer a question that cannot be answered and the 'blame game' is not productive. TB and the isolation experience may have lowered your self-esteem. This is very common. To combat these feelings, try to engage in activities that you know will increase your self-confidence.

You will find that even small household chores such as the washing up can be fulfilling because In isolation, one has to ask for virtually everything that is needed and most tasks have to be done for you. Undertaking chores at home will make you feel that you are in control of your life again.

If you have a job and you are isolated in the community, if possible try to work from home using the telephone or the Internet. If you are unemployed, try continuing with or starting new creative activities. Do not underestimate these benefits.

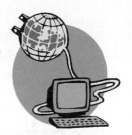

Your psychological well-being is important. It could make the difference between adhering to medication or giving up. It needs to be taken seriously. Speak to your TB specialist about your feelings. He or she might be able to refer you to a clinical psychologist who will help you to understand your feelings and provide you with strategies to deal with them.

Summary

Readers of this book are located in many countries and in some, referral to a dietician or clinical psychologist may not be possible. However, eating as healthily as possible, rest and sleep, and taking exercise should be your goals.

Stigma is being tackled widely but there are still those that perpetuate it. With the understanding and help of nurses and other healthcare providers, TB patients around the world will hopefully feel less like exiles in their own community and more simply just like any other type of patient with a curable disease – the key word being 'curable'.

TB is tackled in different ways all over the world. The services in place to manage and control the disease will differ from region to region. Find out what is available to help you help yourself. Much of what I have written here is complimentary to TB treatment. **The primary key to being cured of the disease is, as always, taking all of the medication.**

Chapter 8

THE GROWING PATIENT MOVEMENT

"Why organize a support network for TB patients? Because we are voiceless, except for the sound of our coughs and groans... do not moan, organize! For the millions that know that TB means suffering, isolation, and stigma – now is the time for action, together."

www.tbtv.org

Since my own experience with MDR-TB in 1995 and the First Edition of *The Tuberculosis Survival Handbook*, much has changed. There is now much more support for people with TB available. In the same year that I was ill, the World Health Organization recommended strategy, DOTS (Directly Observed Therapy, short-course), to control TB was launched. Since then, more than 20 million people have been treated using DOTS and 182 countries have adopted the strategy. Where there are sound DOTS programs operating, it can cure over 85% of detected cases of TB [1]. With the right commitment to the strategy, the DOTS strategy can cure many more. It is increasingly recognized that TB patients have an important role to play in terms of TB control. The engagement and empowerment of patients is now an integral part of the Stop TB strategy to control TB [2].

Nurses play a vital role in this plan. The nurse or other primary health worker may be the first to suspect TB in patients who have been coughing for more than three weeks, or who have not responded to antibiotics, have lost weight or are feeling tired. In some cases, the village volunteer, an extension of the primary health care team into the community, helps TB patients complete their treatment by keeping a regular supply of drugs and assuring they are taken correctly. In urban areas, nurses perform much the tasks as part of DOT.

So how exactly can people with TB get involved in the fight against the disease?

A good example of this is some of the new patient initiatives that we see emerging. Some patients work purely at a local level in their own communities and region. Others are more vocal and have started to make their presence known. Of the latter, tbtv.org is a good example. Created in November 2004, the organization was established by one person. Registered as an NGO (non-governmental organization) and not for profit, it started life as a media platform. Basically, it was a web site where people could share their TB experiences and have a voice. In a short space of time it has grown from one voice to many. As well as raising awareness of the disease, the organization has been instrumental in the development of the Patient's TB Charter, which will be launched on World TB Day 2006 (please see "Useful sources of information for patients"). It has also had a large impact at the international policy level. One cannot go to any important conference on tuberculosis anywhere in the world without meeting someone from tbtv.org.

Personally, this is a wonderful change for me to see. I started my career in the field of HIV activism when the battle against the virus was gaining momentum in the early 1990s and can now see a similar passion with tbtv.org. Passion is a vital ingredient. Over time it can make the difference. It is important because of the affect on us as patients, to have our voices heard and be represented at policy level. We need more organizations such as tbtv.org. I have cited their story simply because it demonstrates that one motivated person can become two and then grow in numbers to collectively start to make a difference. I encourage you to visit their website at www.tbtv.org and see what they are accomplishing. The organization is always willing to work with new people and I am sure that they would like to hear from you.

You do not need an invitation to become involved with TB. If you are passionate about it there are many tasks one can do whether it is preferred to work alone or in a group. You might, perhaps, like to start writing a newsletter for people with TB or you may want to create a website or find other ways to bring people together within this lonely disease. You could also use your story once you are cured of TB to encourage others to complete their treatment. You know how hard it is to take so many tablets everyday, you are an expert on this, what could you do to help other people maintain their treatment?

Other ideas may be to contact your local hospital and offer to write to people who are in isolation with TB. Just being able to communicate with someone who has been through the experience would mean so much to someone who could not leave the room and felt alone.

You could offer to stand-up and be counted (if you are feeling brave!). You could speak to the newspapers, radio and perhaps television about having TB. There is a lot of stigma around the disease. It would help to break it down by talking openly about it. The more people hear about TB, the more that they will understand the disease and the less of a taboo it would be. This may not be for everyone. You may want to volunteer for an already established organization. It does not matter if you feel you have no skills. You have the experience of having tuberculosis and going through treatment. You have an insight to the disease that not many people have. You could lobby for change in you locality, region or country. You could be another voice that adds to the growing demands for more research and development into new diagnostics and treatment options for TB.

The point is that you have had more than TB. You have had a useful experience that can help to control TB in the future. You are a resource and there are people who want to work with you. You simply need to seek them out.

This book is based on my own experience of having been through the TB treatment journey. Many others have successfully been cured of the disease. They too have amazing stories to tell. If you have a story that you would like to share with others you can at *"The Tuberculosis Survival Project"* website. The internet address is **www.tbsurvivalproject.org**

Having HIV changed my life and gave me the impetus to write my first book. Having tuberculosis changed me even more and for the past decade I have worked in the field of this disease; it is what led me to write this book. Without my illnesses I most likely would never had started to write.

I sometimes wonder if having MDR-TB was part of my destiny. It is important for you to think about the future and wonder, perhaps, whether TB is part of your destiny, too. I am sure I will meet some of you in future that have read this book, as part of the ever-growing patient movement that is essential to beating the disease globally. Perhaps I will read the newsletters you write or log onto your website, or sign your new TB organization's petition. Whatever you do, when you have been cured of TB, pass the message on to others. Tell others how you did it, and remind them that they are not alone.

Appendix A

TB-TIPS - ADVICE FOR PATIENTS

- TB is curable - If you feel someone else has exposed you to TB do not panic!

- If you are in contact with someone who has been diagnosed with TB, you should tell your doctor so that he can carry out appropriate tests to see if you need treatment.

- Depending on your personal circumstances, your doctor may feel it is appropriate to put you on medication to prevent you from developing TB - even if you appear uninfected.

- If you develop any such symptoms as: persistent cough, blood stained sputum, fever, night sweats or weight loss, see your doctor immediately for a check-up. The sooner you are treated for TB disease, the sooner you will be cured.

- The symptoms of TB vary from person to person. Any combination of the symptoms mentioned above are worth being checked out.

- Sometimes you will have to wait a long time for test results. It serves no purpose to become stressed during this time. Try to be patient. It will probably be good news.

- If you do not understand what a doctor tells you, ask again... and again, until you do understand. Do not be intimidated by clinicians - they are human, too! Sometimes, because they understand the problem, it is easy for them to assume that you also understand it. Take a notepad if necessary.

- Take a friend with you when you go to see the doctor. It helps to be able to talk over what you have heard with someone you know well. It also helps them to know what is happening to you.

- If tests show that you are latently infected with TB remember you are not infectious; only about 10% of people go on to develop active TB disease. However, if you are immuno-compromised in any way, you may be more at risk. Talk to your doctor about this.

- You may have to spend some time apart from people who may be considered vulnerable. Having to spend time away from friends during a time of need can be hard, but it is a necessary precaution. It is better to ensure they are safe!

- If contact tracing is initiated, disclosing names of people with whom you have been in contact may be embarrassing and awkward. Once again, it is best to be ensure their safety. Conversely, one of the people on your list may have infected you, and may need help and treatment themselves.

- Nurses will welcome talking with you if you need help. They are often easier to communicate with than doctors and are trained to do this as part of their job. They are also generally more approachable.

STORING YOUR MEDICATION

- There are ways of storing medication other than leaving them in their bottles in a shopping bag. Using containers such as a 'dosett' box (plastic wallets that have speared boxes for each day of the week) or 'medimax' (a pill dispenser with compartments that are labeled with days of the week and also the times when pills should be taken) to store each day's supply of drugs, allows you to see if you have taken them as scheduled.

- If you want to store or keep your medicines in a container or pack other than the one the pharmacist has supplied, always check that it is acceptable to use boxes such as those mentioned above. Some drugs need to be stored separately or they could lose their potency.

  If you do take your medicines out of the pharmacy container and place them with other pills, it is best that you only do this with just one day's supply.

- If you cannot get the boxes, try sputum sample containers. Write the days of the week on them, indicating whether this is your morning or evening dose. They can easily be carried around in a handbag or pocket. If you do not want them to rattle, place a little wool in the pot with the pills.

TAKING YOUR MEDICATION

- Taking large quantities of pills may seem physically impossible to some and therefore, one should set aside some time to take them. Taking them quickly may result in nausea and possibly even vomiting. If you have a problem with nausea, tell your TB specialist and he or she may be able to help you. Obviously, if you are vomiting you will not absorb any drug, and the TB may come back.

- Some people find it difficult to remember to take their medication. Try putting your medicine in a prominent place, for example by your coffee or tea in the morning. You might also like to try using an alarm such as a bleeping watch or a computer to help you remember. Encourage a friend or family member to help remind you to take your medication.

- The most important aspect of any drug therapy is forward planning. Always carry an extra dose of medication with you, know when your prescription is due to run out and how to get more pills. If you are going to travel, never keep all of your drugs in a suitcase that will be left in a baggage hold: always carry some extra doses on your person.

- Constantly affirm to yourself that the pills are doing you good, and if you kept taking them regularly, one day you will not need to take them anymore. Believe me when that day comes, you will be glad of your self-discipline.

- It may feel as though your body really is not coping with the pills you are taking. In this case, try taking them with yogurt and a glass of water to help get them down. It seems to make the pills a little more gentle on the stomach.

- If you are a regular (or heavy) alcohol drinker, speak to your doctor about it. It is unlikely to be compatible with the medication you are taking. You may be able to get extra help.

- You may find you develop thrush in your mouth and /or throat. It is a common affliction for people who are immuno-compromised or for those who are taking large amounts of antibiotics for a long period of time.

- You may have thought about trying homeopathic or other alternative therapies on their own. Although these therapies are a useful addition to routine medication, they will not cure you of TB!

- **N.B.** Children with TB pose special problems. Try not to get upset: taking TB medication becomes very routine after awhile but it could be made worse if you and your child fight over it. Try to tempt them using sweets after they had their pills but do not mix the two. You might promise them a big surprise at the end of their treatment. Discuss any problems, such as point blank refusal, with your doctor. Some TB drugs come in syrup form.

- **Keep all medication out of the reach of children.**

DEALING WITH SIDE EFFECTS

• Some of the side effects of medication are very unpleasant such as the older and second-line treatments. I personally needed counseling to get me through and there were many times I sat on the floor in tears surrounded by bottles of pills.

• Doctors are really very good at treating conditions such as TB, though they do not always grasp how side effects make people feel. If your doctor seems unsympathetic, ask to see a counselor or a clinical psychologist. Sometimes they have other ways of dealing with side effects.

• If you are not already on the Direct Observed Therapy program (DOT), ask to be enrolled. This will provide you with much needed emotional and other types of support.

COPING WITH ISOLATION

During the course of isolation you may lose perspective of time. Every day feels the same as the one before, and it may be difficult to determine what happened and when it occurred. This period be very confusing.
To combat this:

• Make sure that people close to you know where you are!

• Is there a clock in the room? If not ask if you can have one or get someone to bring one to you. Ideally, try to get a clock that does not tick. I found that the incessant ticking of the clock eventually drove me 'round the bend' - I ended up pulling it off the wall and smashing it. It never ticked again, but I also did not know the time.

• Try and establish some sort of routine.

- Open your blinds or curtains when you get up, and close them when you go to bed. Sitting in a darkened room may confuse day and night.

- If you are well enough, get up and get dressed.

- If you have a telephone, it will help you greatly. Find out if you are liable for the cost of any calls made and if you do not make any outgoing calls, you can still receive incoming calls at no cost.

- If there is not a telephone in the room, mention it to the staff. It is important to communicate with friends and family, and to maintain contact with the outside world. The staff should understand and be able to help. Remember, if you get this organized, there will be a telephone ready for the next occupant of the room.

- If having your own telephone is a real problem, ask if there is a portable pay phone you can use, which can be brought to your bed. Obviously, this makes receiving incoming calls problematic but ask the nurses if they can take any messages for you and give the details of how to contact you to your friends.

- You may try rearranging the furniture in your room. This helps to personalize it and it may provide you with a certain sense of control.

- If you have a television in your room, try to watch scheduled programs e.g. the news. These will act as regular markers, helping to structure your day.

- Most hospitals have someone who comes around selling newspapers and magazines: make sure you are not left out.

- You may feel that you have lost control over many aspects of your life, but you can still exercise some of the rights that we all enjoy. If you are isolated, there will be warning signs on the outer door telling people what to do when they come in to your room. Make one of your own that says: 'Please knock before you enter.' It is a strange contradiction of isolation, as there is very little privacy. However, it could be embarrassing by being exposed, after a shower for example, when someone, such as a cleaner, needs to enter your room.

- Ask someone to bring some personal effects from home such as pictures or posters. This may help to further personalize what might otherwise feel like an austere little cell.

- Keep a diary, draw, or do some other activity to make the time pass creatively. It is good to feel you are achieving something.

- Some isolation rooms have a facility to make coffee or tea and a fridge so that the occupant can make their own. It is not nice to have to ask for a drink every time you want one and if you feel well enough, it provides a little more independence.

- If you are a smoker and are allowed to smoke (in a negative-pressure room it may be allowed) make sure that you have an ample supplies of cigarettes. For smokers, it is difficult to get through the day with no cigarettes if no one is going to visit, and the demon of addiction starts to nag!

- If you are to be isolated for awhile, you are going to need clean clothes. Ask the nurses if they can do the wash for you. There are usually facilities for doing this but make sure you mark your clothes in some way so that they can be identified.

- If you have some space in your room, you may feel like doing a little exercise. Ask whether you can see the physiotherapist. He or she may be able to provide some equipment and/or advice. Isolation compounded with the weight loss due to the TB leads to muscle wasting. Try to keep some muscle tone.

- Ask to see a psychologist regularly if you are having trouble with the combination of isolation and side effects. Frustration, resentment and loss of control are common feelings, and they may be able to help you deal with them.

- Remember, you are undergoing treatment. At times it may seem hard, but a relatively short time of discomfort could ensure a complete return to health.

- Try to make an effort with you personal appearance. It is important for self-esteem.

- Fluorescent lighting gives some people headaches. You should be able to bring in a bedside lamp or other lighting from home.

DIET

- It is possible to eat well on a budget, but it can be difficult. One needs motivation and you have to know what to buy. Buy a lot of fresh foods regularly and shop around! Do not just go to your local super market as they may charge more and the food may not be as fresh as that from a specialist store. It is easy to get distracted in supermarkets by less nutritious convenience food. If you have a freezer, try cooking in bulk. This is very cost-effective.

- Eating foods high in vitamin B12 may help prevent TB. These include: Meat, Fish, Eggs, Dairy Products, Wholegrain Cereals, Beans, Wheatgerm,

Green Vegetables, Yeast Extracts, Fortified Breakfast Cereals, Grapenuts, Branflakes (check label), some Soya milks.

• After a period of illness and/or isolation, you may want to go drinking with your friends. Being able to socialize again will feel wonderful. However, high alcohol intake after a period of weakness may affect your body's repair mechanisms. Alcohol has no nutritional value and gives a false sense of energy. It can affect your appetite and lower the levels of vitamins in your body. Remember, a regular high intake may also adversely affect the regularity with which you take your medication.

• **If you have got any questions ask a dietician!**

Appendix B

YOUR PERSONAL TB TREATMENT CHART

The following charts are for the purpose of logging every dose of treatment that you take. The charts cover a period of nine months. It is possible that you will only need to take treatment for six. Write the names of the drugs that you are taking and date in the appropriate boxes. Tick the boxes each time you take your TB medication.

Remember:

• There is no secret to surviving tuberculosis; it is simply about taking every dose of medication.

• Tell your TB specialist if you are having problems taking your medication or experiencing side effects.

• Only to stop when you are told to do so by a TB specialist.

NAME OF TABLET	WEEK 1							WEEK 2							WEEK 3							WEEK 4						
	M	T	W	T	F	S	S	M	T	W	T	F	S	S	M	T	W	T	F	S	S	M	T	W	T	F	S	S

NAME OF TABLET	WEEK 1							WEEK 2							WEEK 3							WEEK 4						
	M	T	W	T	F	S	S	M	T	W	T	F	S	S	M	T	W	T	F	S	S	M	T	W	T	F	S	S

NAME OF TABLET	WEEK 1							WEEK 2							WEEK 3							WEEK 4						
	M	T	W	T	F	S	S	M	T	W	T	F	S	S	M	T	W	T	F	S	S	M	T	W	T	F	S	S

NAME OF TABLET	WEEK 1							WEEK 2							WEEK 3							WEEK 4						
	M	T	W	T	F	S	S	M	T	W	T	F	S	S	M	T	W	T	F	S	S	M	T	W	T	F	S	S

NAME OF TABLET	WEEK 1							WEEK 2							WEEK 3							WEEK 4						
	M	T	W	T	F	S	S	M	T	W	T	F	S	S	M	T	W	T	F	S	S	M	T	W	T	F	S	S

NAME OF TABLET	WEEK 1							WEEK 2							WEEK 3							WEEK 4						
	M	T	W	T	F	S	S	M	T	W	T	F	S	S	M	T	W	T	F	S	S	M	T	W	T	F	S	S

NAME OF TABLET	WEEK 1							WEEK 2							WEEK 3							WEEK 4						
	M	T	W	T	F	S	S	M	T	W	T	F	S	S	M	T	W	T	F	S	S	M	T	W	T	F	S	S

NAME OF TABLET	WEEK 1							WEEK 2							WEEK 3							WEEK 4						
	M	T	W	T	F	S	S	M	T	W	T	F	S	S	M	T	W	T	F	S	S	M	T	W	T	F	S	S

NAME OF TABLET	WEEK 1							WEEK 2							WEEK 3							WEEK 4						
	M	T	W	T	F	S	S	M	T	W	T	F	S	S	M	T	W	T	F	S	S	M	T	W	T	F	S	S

GLOSSARY

Acid-fast bacilli (AFB): *bacteria of the genus of Mycobacteria:* it is called acid-fast because of its staining properties in diagnostic tests in the laboratory.

Active Tuberculosis: currently active tuberculosis disease, whether or not it is infectious.

Bacilli: rod-shaped bacteria.

Bacteria: group of micro-organisms, which lack a distinctive nuclear membrane and are considered more primitive than plant or animal cells. Most bacteria are unicellular (consisting of only one cell). Bacteria reproduces by dividing itself. Bacteria can be spherical, rod-shaped, spiral or corkscrew-shaped. They are present virtually everywhere. Some of them are harmless - others are very dangerous.

Bacterium: singular of the above definition of bacteria.

BCG: Bacille Calmette-Guerin, the vaccine currently used to prevent tuberculosis, named after the scientists who discovered it.

CDC: Center for Disease Control and Prevention, Atlanta, USA.

Closed tuberculosis: tuberculosis that is not active.

Culture: to grow under laboratory conditions over time.

Directly Observed Therapy (DOT): Supervised therapy in which, a responsible person, usually a nurse, watches the patient take every dose of treatment and reports if any doses are missed.

Drug-resistant tuberculosis: Tuberculosis, which is resistant to one or more anti-tuberculosis drugs.

First line anti-tuberculosis drugs: rifampicin, isoniazid, pyramzinamide, Ethambutol, and streptomycin.

Heaf Test: commonly used skin test in which 'tuberculin' is injected with a multiple puncture apparatus. After a period of time a positive result indicates the presence of TB. However, this test result can only be interpreted by a health care professional. It is complicated to read and a positive result does not necessarily mean that one has tuberculosis.

HIV related tuberculosis: tuberculosis in an HIV-infected individual (tuberculosis is now an AIDS-defining disease).

Latent tuberculosis (sometimes known as 'dormant tuberculosis'): a state in which viable mycobacteria (the bacteria that causes tuberculosis) are present in the body without currently causing active disease but with the potential to activate and cause disease.

Mantoux Test: The Mantoux test is used in the United States and is endorsed by the American Thoracic Society and the CDC. It is very similar in principle to the Heaf test, with the exception that a single injection site is made into the skin in the same place as the Heaf test. A stronger strength of tuberculin PPD is used and a result can be measured after 48-72 hours to grade a positive or negative result [3].

MDR-TB: Multidrug-resistant tuberculosis is a form of TB that is resistant to two or more of the primary drugs used to treat tuberculosis.

Mycobacterium tuberculosis: the bacterium that causes tuberculosis.

Negative: not affirming the presence of an organism or condition when looked for i.e., a negative diagnosis.

Negative Pressure Room: a special room where the air pressure is lower than outside the room.

Old / Previous Tuberculosis: tuberculosis disease which has either healed naturally or been fully treated and shows no evidence of current activity. It may or may not be 'latent'.

Open Tuberculosis: see tuberculosis disease and sputum smear positive tuberculosis.

Positive: indicates the presence of an organism or condition and provides a positive diagnosis.

Reactivated tuberculosis: old tuberculosis infection (whether previously known or not) which has become active.

Re-infection: active tuberculosis due to acquisition of new infection in someone who has had previous tuberculosis infection.

Smear: in the case of tuberculosis diagnosis and monitoring, this means that acid fast bacilli (mentioned above) are clearly present without culture.

Sputum: matter ejected from the lungs, bronchi and trachea and out though the mouth, i.e.phlegm.

Sputum Smear Positive Tuberculosis: (sometimes still called 'open' tuberculosis): pulmonary tuberculosis in which mycobacteria ('acid-fast bacilli, AFB) have been stained in a smear of sputum and examined under a microscope.

Stain / Staining: the use of dye for producing coloration in tissues or micro-organisms for microscopic examination.

Supervised Therapy: treatment which is closely supervised by the designated tuberculosis physician working with the TB nurse specialist or equivalent. In the community, 'supervised therapy' implied and adherence to treatment will be monitored at least monthly, but the patient will not normally be observed to take the treatment (see also Directly Observed Therapy).

TB Nurse Specialist: the nurse, ideally with special training in tuberculosis and one who has responsibility for tuberculosis services in the community. The nurse will normally, but not necessarily, work from the chest clinic. A variety of other titles are used for nurses doing this work and they are vital to the diagnosis, treatment and surveillance of TB and MDR-TB.

T-SPOT.*TB* test: A blood test that detects the T-cells in the blood. TB infection induces a strong response by immune cells in the bood called 'T-cells'.

Tuberculin Skin Test (TST): see Heaf test, Manteaux test.

Tuberculosis (TB): infectious disease caused by the *Mycobacterium tuberculosis*.

Tuberculosis Infection: a condition in which tuberculosis organisms are present in the body without necessarily evidence of tuberculosis disease.

+++; *see 'Positive' above:* In terms of medical test results it indicates either a low, medium or high amount of organisms present depending on how many positives there are in the result. Three positives result is the highest.

+/- : can be described as 'scanty' or negligible, not quite warranting one whole +.

USEFUL SOURCES OF INFORMATION FOR PATIENTS

PART 1:

THE WORLD CARE COUNCIL: PATIENTS' RIGHTS AND RESPONSIBILITIES

On World TB Day 2006 the Patients charter was launched. The newly formed World Care Council was the driving force behind the document. It is a patient driven effort and reflects the growing reality that people with TB are being seen more as partners in the control of the disease rather than merely patients.

Powered by people from around the globe concerned by six million avoidable deaths a year, the World Care Council, a non-governmental organization, has been established to turn worthy words and medical recommendations into life-saving realities.

The World Care Council aims to improve the quality of care for people with Tuberculosis, HIV/AIDS, and Malaria, by bringing people with the diseases and health professionals together in a global health initiative to raise the standards of care. By developing patient-centered standards of rights, responsibilities and recommendations for each the three diseases, such as the Patients' Charter (reproduced below) and it's tandem International Standards, with implementation and monitoring programs in affected communities, the World Care Council is forging new tools for the fight against the world's pandemics.

www.worldcarecouncil.org

The Patients' Charter for Tuberculosis Care

The Patients' Charter outlines the Rights and Responsibilities of People with Tuberculosis. It empowers people with the disease and their communities through this knowledge. Initiated and developed by patients from around the world, the Charter makes the relationship with health care providers a mutually beneficial one.

The Charter sets out the ways in which patients, the community, health providers, both private and public, and governments can work as partners in a positive and open relationship with a view to improving tuberculosis care and enhancing the effectiveness of the health care process. It allows for all parties to be held more accountable to each other, fostering mutual interaction and a 'positive partnership'.

Developed in tandem with the *International Standards for Tuberculosis Care*[1] to promote a 'patient-centered' approach, the Charter bears in mind the principles on health and human rights of the United Nations, UNESCO, WHO, Council of Europe, as well as other local and national charters and conventions[2].

The Patients Charter for Tuberculosis Care practices the principle of Greater Involvement of People with TB. This affirms that the empowerment of people with the disease is the catalyst for effective collaboration with health providers and authorities, and is essential to victory in the fight to stop TB. The Patients' Charter, the first global 'patient-powered' standard for care, is a cooperative tool, forged from common cause, for the entire TB Community.

Patients' Rights

1. Care
   a. The right to free and equitable access to tuberculosis care, from diagnosis through treatment completion, regardless of resources, race, gender, age, language, legal status, religious beliefs, sexual orientation, culture or having another illness.
   b. The right to receive medical advice and treatment which fully meets the new International Standards for Tuberculosis Care, centering on patient needs, including those with MDR-TB or TB-HIV coinfections, and preventative treatment for young children and others considered to be at high risk.
   c. The right to benefit from proactive health sector community outreach, education and prevention campaigns as part of comprehensive care programs.

2. Dignity
   a. The right to be treated with respect and dignity, including the delivery of services without stigma, prejudice or discrimination by health providers and authorities.
   b. The right to quality health care in a dignified environment, with moral support from family, friends and the community.

3. Information
   a. The right to information about what health care services are available for tuberculosis, and what responsibilities, engagements, and direct or indirect costs, are involved.
   b. The right to receive a timely, concise and clear description of the medical condition, with diagnosis, prognosis (an opinion as to the likely future course of the illness), and treatment proposed, with communication of common risks and appropriate alternatives.

    c.   *The right to know the names and dosages of any medication or intervention to be prescribed, its normal actions and potential side-effects, and its possible impact on other conditions or treatments.*

    d.   *The right of access to medical information which relates to the patient's condition and treatment, and a copy of the medical record if requested by the patient or a person autthorized by the patient.*

    e.   *The right to meet, share experiences with peers and other patients, and to voluntary counseling at any time from diagnosis through treatment completion.*

4. Choice

    a.   *The right to a second medical opinion, with access to previous medical records.*

    b.   *The right to accept or refuse surgical interventions if chemotherapy is possible, and to be informed of the likely medical and statutory consequences within the context of a communicable disease.*

    c.   *The right to choose whether or not to take part in research programs without compromising care.*

5. Confidence

    a.   *The right to have personal privacy, dignity, religious beliefs and culture respected.*

    b.   *The right to have information relating to the medical condition kept confidential, and released to other authorities contingent upon the patient's consent.*

6. Justice

    a.   *The right to make a complaint through channels provided for this purpose by the health authority, and to have any complaint dealt with promptly and fairly.*

   b. *The right to appeal to a higher authority if the above is not respected, and to be informed in writing of the outcome.*

7. Organization

   a. *The right to join, or to establish, organizations of people with or affected by tuberculosis, and to seek support for the development of these clubs and community based associations through the health providers, authorities, and civil society.*

   b. *The right to participate as 'stakeholders' in the development, implementation, monitoring and evaluation of TB policies and programs with local, national and international health authorities.*

8. Security

   a. *The right to job security after diagnosis or appropriate rehabilitation upon completion of treatment.*

   b. *The right to nutritional security or food supplements if needed to meet treatment requirements.*

Patients' Responsibilities

1. Share Information

   a. *The responsibility to provide the health care giver as much information as possible about present health, past illnesses, any allergies and any other relevant details.*

   b. *The responsibility to provide information to the health provider about contacts with immediate family, friends and others who may be vulnerable to tuberculosis or may have been infected by contact.*

2. Follow Treatment
   a. The responsibility to follow the prescribed and agreed treatment plan, and to conscientiously comply with the instructions given to protect the patient's health, and that of others.
   b. The responsibility to inform the health provider of any difficulties or problems with following treatment, or if any part of the treatment is not clearly understood.

3. Contribute to Community Health
   a. The responsibility to contribute to community well being by encouraging others to seek medical advice if they exhibit the symptoms of tuberculosis.
   b. The responsibility to show consideration for the rights of other patients and health care providers, understanding that this is the dignified basis and respectful foundation of the TB Community.

4. Solidarity
   a. The moral responsibility of showing solidarity with other patients, marching together towards cure.
   b. The moral responsibility to share information and knowledge gained during treatment, and to pass this expertise to others in the community, making empowerment contagious.
   c. The moral responsibility to join in efforts to make the community TB Free.

Help turn these words into realities. Support the drive towards implementation in the community. sign on-line at **http://www.wcc-tb.org** or sign-up by SMS text: +33 679 486 024. In common cause, with mutual respect, together we can raise the standards of care.

1. International Standards for Tuberculosis Care:
   http://www.worldcarecouncil.org/pdf/
2. United Nations CESCR General Comment 14 on the right to health:
   http://www.worldcarecouncil.org/pdf/
   - WHO Ottawa Charter on health promotion:
     http://www.worldcarecouncil.org/pdf/
   - The Council of Europe Convention for the Protection of Human
     Rights and Dignity/ biology and medicine:
     http://www.worldcarecouncil.org/pdf/
   - UNESCO Universal Draft Declaration on Bioethics and Human
     Rights: **http://www.worldcarecouncil.org/pdf/**

Comments warmly welcome: **voices@wcc-tb.org**
version pdf: **http://www.worldcarecouncil.org/pdf/**
Thanks to the American Thoracic Society (**www.thoracic.org**) and the
Open Society Institute (**www.soros.org**) for their support Patients'
Charter for Tuberculosis Care.

© **2006 World Care Council / Conseil Mondial de Soins**

PART 2:
OTHER SOURCES OF INFORMATION

American Lung Association – wwwlungusa.org

The mission of the American Lung Association® is to prevent lung disease and promote lung health.

The American Lung Association® is the oldest voluntary health organization in the United States, with a National Office and constituent and affiliate associations around the country. Founded in 1904 to fight tuberculosis, the American Lung Association® today fights lung disease in all its forms, with special emphasis on asthma, tobacco control and environmental health. The American Lung Association® is funded by contributions from the public, along with gifts and grants from corporations, foundations and government agencies. The American Lung Association® achieves its many successes through the work of thousands of committed volunteers and staff.

The Stop TB Partnership – www.stoptb.org

The Stop TB Partnership was established in 2000 to realize the goal of eliminating TB as a public health problem and, ultimately, to obtain a world free of TB. It comprises a network of international organizations, countries, donors from the public and private sectors, governmental and non-governmental organizations and individuals that have expressed an interest in working together to achieve this goal.

TB Alert – www.tbalert.co.uk

TB Alert is the UK's National and International Tuberculosis charity - the only British charity working solely on fighting TB in the UK and overseas.

TB Alert is a young charity, registered in late 1998 and launched at the Houses of Parliament on World TB Day (24th March) 1999. It was set up by people who felt that with its long tradition of TB work, there should be a greater response in Britain to the resurgent threat of tuberculosis - already declared a global emergency by the World Health Organization (WHO) in 1993.

TB Alert is the first TB-specific charity in Britain since the 1960s when earlier organizations, assuming too soon that the disease had been vanquished, faded away or moved on to other interests. It operates almost entirely on the time and energy of volunteers, with its first employee only starting in November 2001. Its active Trustees include many of the leading experts on TB based in Britain

TBTV – www.tbtv.org

We are a group of patients, former patients, health professionals and concerned 'global citizens' who have recognized both the complete lack of support for the millions of people who suffer from tuberculosis, and the silence and stigma that permit this deadly epidemic to increase its carnage each year.

We believe that this must change, and that we must act now.

To bring together many other folks from around the world into a dynamic network, we have set up a non-profit, non-governmental organization which is registered in France as an Association (1901). This structure allows for the direct participation of many individuals, and for the development of relationships and partnerships with a wide variety of institutions, organizations and enterprises.

The Tuberculosis Survival Project – www.tbsurvivalproject.org

As a result of this book, *The Tuberculosis Survival Project* was formed. The aim of the project is to create a platform where people can tell their own stories of having TB. The disease has influenced many of the great writers in the past such as the Brönte sisters, John Keats, Katherine Mansfield and George Orwell. The project is about capturing that same essence of these great writers. What separates these "old consumptives" and people who have the disease today is that there is effective treatment. Tuberculosis is a curable disease where drugs are available and treatment is adhered to. This project encourages people to write about their own experience of TB/MDR-TB. In the future it is hoped that these works will be collected together to become a book called *"Tuberculosis in the 21st Century – A People's Diary"*. If you wish to share your story with others then you can email it to mystory@tbsurvivalproject.org

World Economic Forum – Global Health Initiative - A TB Awareness Building Toolkit for Professionals

http://www.weforum.org/site/homepublic.nsf/Content/Global+Health+Initiative%5CTools+for+Business

This Awareness Building Tuberculosis/Multidrug-resistant tuberculosis (MDR-TB) Toolkit has been developed by the Global Health Initiative of the World Economic Forum, with the support of Eli Lilly and in partnership with the International Council of Nurses. It is especially designed to support companies that are starting to implement TB workplace programs and those with existing programs.

There are 8,000,000 new TB cases, 2,000,000 deaths and an estimated 400,000 new cases of MDR-TB around the world every year. Yet TB can be treated and cured. The internationally recognized strategy for TB control – the DOTS strategy – has proven remarkably effective. The World Bank has described the Directly Observed Treatment Short-course DOTS strategy as one of the "most cost-effective of all health interventions". Encouragingly, businesses in different countries have started to implement TB control and DOTS programs in their workplaces; however, one common challenge they face is how to increase employee awareness of TB and how to educate workers and health staff on the symptoms of TB and treatment possibilities.

This toolkit aims to help companies in this situation – it is a ready-to-use toolkit that can allow companies to raise staff's awareness of TB and how to treat it effectively. The toolkit is meant for: Managers who aim to implement TB workplace programs; Healthcare professionals, e.g., physicians, nurses and allied health professionals, who should have a good knowledge of TB; Employees who are infected with TB. Materials in the toolkit can help you: 1) Raise general employee awareness of TB and its symptoms 2) Support TB patients at work 3) Provide information on TB for human resources departments, healthcare professionals (e.g., physicians, nurses and allied health professionals) and other care and support staff 4) Provide constant reminders to company employees about key facts through the poster and leaflets included in this kit.

REFERENCES

Introduction

1. *World Health Organization, Guidelines for the Management of Drug-Resistant Tuberculosis, (WHO/CDS/TB/2005.XXX), World Health Organization, Geneva, Switzerland.*

2. *DeAngelis CD, Flanagin A. Tuberculosis – a global problem requiring a global solution. JAMA. 2005;293:2793-2794*

3. *Dye, C (2005), Global TB epidemiology and progress towards the Millennium Development Goals. Joint Meeting of the DOTS Expansion, TB/HIV and DOTS-Plus Working Groups in Memory of Lisa Veron, Symposium of the 36th World Conference on Lung Health, Paris, France, 18 October 2005.*

Chapter 1

1. *World Health Organization (2006). Global tuberculosis control: surveillance, planning, financing. WHO report 2006. Geneva: WHO/HTM/TB/2006.362.*

2. *Styblo K (1967). Epidemiological and clinical study of Tuberculosis in the district of Kolin, Czechoslovakia. Bull World Health Organization 37: 819-874*

3. *World Health Organization (2004). Treatment of Tuberculosis: Guidelines for National Programs, 3rd edition, revised Geneva: WHO/CDS/TB 2003.313/rev.*

4. *Jaramillo E (1999). Encompassing prevention with treatment: the path for a lasting control of tuberculosis, Social Science & Medicine, 49: 393-404.*

5. *Dye C (2005). Global TB epidemiology and progress toward the Millenium Development Goals. Joint Meeting of the DOTS Expansion, TB/HIV and DOTS-Plus Workng Groups in Memory of Lisa Veron. Symposium of the 36th World Conference on Lung Health, Paris, France, 18 October 2005.*

6. *The WHO/IUATLD global project on anti-tuberculosis drug resistance surveillance (2004). Anti-tuberculosis drug resistance in the world: third global report, 1999–2002. World Health Organization, Geneva: WHO/HTM/TB/2004.343.*

7. Geerligs, W.A., van Altena, R., de Lange, W.C, M., et al, (2000). Multidrug-resistant tuberculosis: long-term treatment outcome in The Netherlands. Int J Tuberc Lung Dis 2:499-505.

8. Mahmoudi, A., Iseman M,D., (1993). Pitfalls in the care of patients with tuberculosis: common errors and their association with the acquisition of drug resistance. JAMA 270:65-68.

9. Suarez, P. G., K. Floyd, J. Portocarrero, et al., (2002). Feasibility and cost-effectiveness of standardised second-line drug treatment for chronic tuberculosis patients: a national cohort study in Peru. The Lancet. 359:1980-89.

10. Leimane, V., Riekstina, V., Holtz T,H., et al., (2005). Clinical outcome of individualised treatment of multidrug-resistant tuberculosis in Latvia: a retrospective cohort study. The Lancet. 365:318-326

11. Public-private mix for DOTS: report of the second meeting of the PPM subgroup for DOTS expansion (2004). Geneva: WHO/HTM/TB/2004.338. http://whqlibdoc.who.int/hq/2004/WHO_HTM_TB_2004.338.pdf (accessed 11 Jan 2005).

12. PK Dewan, SS Lal, K Lonnroth, et al, Improving tuberculosis control through public-private collaboration in India: literature review. BMJ, doi:10.1136/bmj.38738.473252.7C (published 8 February 2006).

13. World Health Organization/Stop TB Partnership. A guide to monitoring and evaluation for collaborative TB/HIV activities. Geneva: WHO/HTM/TB/2004.342

14. Stop TB Partnership and World Health Organization. Global Plan to Stop TB 2006-2015 (2006). Geneva: WHO/HTM/STB/2006.35

Chapter 2

1. Coker, R.J, From Chaos to Coercion, (2000), p4, St Martins Press, New York.

Chapter 3

Opening quote; World Health Organization (1998), Global Tuberculosis Program, Press Release, Tuberculosis Fact Sheet, Geneva, Switzerland.

1. Blacks Medical Dictionary (1998), 38th Edition, Edited by G. Macpherson MB BS, p342, A & C Black, London.

2. CDC (1994), Questions and Answers about TB, US Health Department of Health and Human Services, p1, USA.

3. World Health Organization (1998), Global Tuberculosis Program, Press Release, Tuberculosis Fact Sheet, Geneva, Switzerland.

4. Marais, F (1998), TB Network Newsletter, A Historical Perspective, TB Network Newsletter (December), p3, TB Network Association, London, United Kingdom.

5. Ryan, F (1992), Tuberculosis: The Greatest Story Never Told, Part 1, p6, Swift Publishers, England.

6. NJMS, National Tuberculosis Center (1996), Brief History of Tuberculosis, USA.

7. Reeder, H.L, Epidemiologic Basis of Tuberculosis Control (1999), p17, International Union Against Tuberculosis and Lung Disease, Paris, France.

8. http://www.euro.who.int/eprise/main/who/progs/tub/20040303_2

9. Marais, F (1998), TB Network Newsletter, A Historical Perspective, TB Network Newsletter (December), p3, TB Network Association, London, United Kingdom.

10. Karlen, A (1996), Plagues Progress, A Social History of Man and Disease An Epidemic of Epidemics, ch1, p5, Indigo, London, United Kingdom.

11. Garret, L (1994), The Coming Plague, p11, Penguin, New York, USA.

12. Karlen, A (1996), Plagues Progress, A Social History of Man and Disease, An Epidemic of Epidemics, ch12, p211, Indigo, London, United Kingdom.

13. The Independent Working Group on Tuberculosis (1998), The Prevention and Control of Tuberculosis in the United Kingdom, UK Guidance of the Prevention and Control of Transmission of 1) HIV-related Tuberculosis, 2) Drug-resistant, Including Multiple Drug-resistant, Tuberculosis. p5, Department of Health, London, United Kingdom.

14. Garret, L (1994), The Coming Plague, p620, Penguin, New York, USA.

15. Karlen, A (1996), Plagues Progress, A Social History of Man and Disease, An Epidemic of Epidemics, ch1, p1, Indigo, London, United Kingdom.

16. World Health Organization (1998), Global Tuberculosis Program, Press Release, Tuberculosis Fact Sheet, Geneva, Switzerland.

17. CDC TB Surveillance Report 2003

18. World Health Organization (1998), Global Tuberculosis Program, Press Release, Tuberculosis Fact Sheet, Geneva, Switzerland.

19. World Health Organization (1998), Global Tuberculosis Program, Press Release, Tuberculosis Fact Sheet, Geneva, Switzerland.

20. Rieder, H.L, Epidemiologic Basis of Tuberculosis Control (1999), p12, International Union Against Tuberculosis and Lung Disease, Paris, France.

21. Understanding Tuberculosis, (2001), (video), London Borough of Newham, London, United Kingdom.

22. Rieder, H.L, Epidemiologic Basis of Tuberculosis Control (1999), p13, International Union Against Tuberculosis and Lung Disease, Paris, France.

23. Rieder, H.L, Epidemiologic Basis of Tuberculosis Control (1999), p11, International Union Against Tuberculosis and Lung Disease, Paris, France.

24. Rieder, H.L, Epidemiologic Basis of Tuberculosis Control (1999), p13, International Union Against Tuberculosis and Lung Disease, Paris, France.

25. The Independent Working Group on Tuberculosis (1998), The Prevention and Control of Tuberculosis in the United Kingdom, UK Guidance of the Prevention and Control of Transmission of 1) HIV-related Tuberculosis, 2) Drug-resistant, Including Multiple Drug-resistant, Tuberculosis. p5, Department of Health, London, United Kingdom.

26. Mayho P, Grice S, Morris S (1996), Positive Carers - The Rights and Responsibilities of HIV Positive Health Care Workers, p3, Cassell PLC, London, United Kingdom.

27. Fitzgerald, John Mark; Grzybowski, Stephan; Allen, Edward, A (1991) Chest, July, v100 n1 p191 (10), The Impact of Human Immuno-deficiency Virus Infection on Tuberculosis and its control, American College of Chest Physicians, USA.

28. WHO. Issues relating to the use of BCG in immunization programmes. A discussion document (unpublished document WHO/V&B/99.23; available from Vaccines and Biologicals, World Health Organization, 1211 Geneva 27, Switzerland.

Chapter 4

Opening Quote; Anon, Ministry of Health (1942)

1. *Stop TB Partnership (2005), The Global Plan to Stop TB 2006-2015, Geneva, Switzerland.*

2. *Coker R.J, (1998), TB Network, Issue 1, p6, TB Network Association, London, United Kingdom.*

3. *CDC (1994), Core Curriculum on Tuberculosis; What the Clinician Should Know, (Third Edition), p19, US Department of Health and Human Services, USA.*

4. *Blacks Medical Dictionary (1998), 38th Edition, Edited by G. Macpherson MB BS, p221, A & C Black, London, United Kingdom.*

5. *CDC (1994), Core Curriculum on Tuberculosis; What the Clinician Should Know, (Third Edition), p27, US Department of Health and Human Services, USA.*

6. *Rothel, R.S, Anderson, P, Diagnosis of Latent Mycobacterium Tuberculosis Infection: is the demise of the Mantoux test imminent?, Future Drugs, 10.1586/14787210.3.6.981, p982, 2005).*

7. *Meier,T., Eulenbruch, H.-P, Wrighton-Smith,P., Enders, G., Regnath, T., (2005), Sensitivity of a new commercial enzyme-linked immunospot assay (T SPOT-TB) for diagnosis of tuberculosis in clinical practice, Eur J Clin Microbiol Infect Dis, 24:529-536, DOI 10.1007/s10096-005-1377-8, (Published online: 19 August 2005), Springer-Verlag.*

8. *Zellweger, J-P., Zellweger, A., Ansermer, S., de Senarclens, B., Wrighton-Smith, P., (2005), Contact tracing using a new T-cell-based test: better correlation with tuberculosis exposure than the tuberculin skin test, Int J Tuberc Lung Dis 9(11):1242-1247.*

9. *Rothel, J,S. Andersen, P (2005),Diagnosis of latent Mycobacterium Tuberculosis Infection: is the demise of the Mantoux test imminent?, Future Drugs, 10.1586/14787210.3.6.981, p988, United Kingdom.*

10. *CDC (1994), Core Curriculum on Tuberculosis; What the Clinician Should Know, (Third Edition), p27, US Department of Health and Human Services, USA.*

11. CDC (1994), Core Curriculum on Tuberculosis; What Clinician's Should Know, (Third Edition), p29, US Department of Health and Human Services, USA.

12. Blacks Medical Dictionary (1998), 38th Edition, edited by G. Macpherson MB BS, p361, A&C Black, London, United Kingdom.

13. The Independent Working Group on Tuberculosis (1998), The Prevention and Control of Tuberculosis in the United Kingdom, Recommendations for the Prevention and Control of Tuberculosis at Local Level, p24, para 15.2, Department of Health, London, United Kingdom.

Chapter 5

Opening quote: Persius (Antus Persius Flaccus) AD34-62, Satires no3, 1.64, Cf Ovid 503:3, The Oxford Dictionary of Quotations, Revised Fourth Edition, Edited by Angela Partington, Oxford University Press (1996), p197.

1. Blacks Medical Dictionary (1998), 38th Edition, edited by G. Macpherson MB BS, p530, A&C Black, London, United Kingdom.

2. Rothel, J,S. Andersen, P (2005),Diagnosis of latent Mycobacterium Tuberculosis Infection: is the demise of the Mantoux test imminent?, Future Drugs, 10.1586/14787210.3.6.981, p982, United Kingdom.

3. Espinal, M,A, (2003),The Global Situation of MDR-TB, Tuberculosis 83, 44-51, Elesevier Science Ltd.

4. Rothel, J,S. Andersen, P (2005),Diagnosis of latent Mycobacterium Tuberculosis Infection: is the demise of the Mantoux test imminent?, Future Drugs, 10.1586/14787210.3.6.981, p982, United Kingdom.

5. World Health Organization, Guidelines for the Management of Drug-Resistant Tuberculosis, (WHO/CDS/TB/2005.xxx), Geneva, Switzerland.

6. Espinal, M.A, The Global Situation of MDR-TB, www.elsevierhealth.com/journals.com/ jounals/tube, Tuberculosis, (2003), 83,44-51.

6. Espinal, M.A, The Global Situation of MDR-TB, www.elsevierhealth.com/journals.com/ jounals/tube, Tuberculosis, (2003), 83,44-51.

7. Espinal, M.A, The Global Situation of MDR-TB, www.elsevierhealth.com/journals.com/ jounals/tube, Tuberculosis, (2003), 83,44-51.

8. World Health Organization, Guidelines for the Management of Drug-Resistant Tuberculosis, (WHO/CDS/TB/2005.xxx), Geneva, Switzerland

9. Gupta et al, Responding to Market Failures, Science Magazine, Vol 293, 10 August 2001.

10. World Health Organization, Instructions for Applying to the Green Light Committee for Access to Second-Line Anti-Tuberculosis Drugs, (WHO/CDS/TB/2001.286 Rev 1), Geneva, Switzerland.

11. CDC (1994), Questions and Answers about TB, US Health Department of Health and Human Services, p10, USA.

12. CDC (1994), Core Curriculum on Tuberculosis; What the Clinician Should Know, (Third Edition), p41, US Department of Health and Human Services, USA.

13. TB Network (1998), Issue 1, p8, TB Network Association, London, United Kingdom.

14. TB Network (1998), Issue 1, p8, TB Network Association, London

15. Bacon, Francis (1625), "Essays of Friendship"

16. Thorax (1994), Control and Prevention of Tuberculosis in the United Kingdom: Code of Practice, p1199, British Thoracic Society, United Kingdom.

17. World Health Organization (1998), Global Tuberculosis Programme, Press Release, Tuberculosis Fact Sheet, Geneva, Switzerland.

18. World Health Organization (1998), Global Tuberculosis Programme, Press Release, Tuberculosis Fact Sheet, Geneva, Switzerland.

Chapter 6

Opening quote: Jeanne Marie Laskas, a writer for The Washington Post. Quote found in the June 1998 edition of Readers Digest.

1. CDC (1994), Questions and Answers about TB, p9, US Department of Health and Human Services, USA.

2. NJMS National Tuberculosis Center (1996), A Brief History of Tuberculosis, USA.

3. Coenson C. MD, Dimsdale J.E. MD. (1994), Psychiatric Liaison on a Bone Marrow Transplant Unit, General Hospital Psychiatry, p131-134, New York, USA.

4. *Coenson C. MD, Dimsdale J.E. MD. (1994), Psychiatric Liaison on a Bone Marrow Transplant Unit, General Hospital Psychiatry, p131, New York, USA.*

5. *Coenson C. MD, Dimsdale J.E. MD. (1994), Psychiatric Liaison on a Bone Marrow Transplant Unit, General Hospital Psychiatry, p131, New York, USA.*

6. *Coenson C. MD, Dimsdale J.E. MD. (1994), Psychiatric Liaison on a Bone Marrow Transplant Unit, General Hospital Psychiatry, p131, New York, USA.*

Chapter 7

Opening quote; Anton Chekov, The Three Sisters (1901) act 4, (translated by Elisaveta Fen), The Oxford Dictionary of Quotations, Revised Fourth Edition, Edited by Angela Partington, Oxford University Press, (1996), p197.

1. *Foods that Harm, Foods that Heal (1997), Readers Digest, Fourth Imprint with amendments, Edited and designed by 'The Readers Digest Association Limited', Editors; Alasdair McWhirter and Liz Classen, p351, United Kingdom.*

Chapter 8

Opening Quote; www.tbtv.org

1. *World Health Organization, (2005), Guidelines for the Management of Drug-Resistant Tuberculosis, (WHO/CDS/TB/2005.XXX), Geneva, Switzerland.*

2. *The Stop TB Strategy (2005), Building on and enhancing DOTS to meet the TB-related millennium development goals, DRAFT PAPER - TO BE PUBLISHED JANUARY 2006, Geneva, Switzerland.*

INDEX